USING YOUR WEIGHTS FOR
WEIGHT LOSS

USING YOUR WEIGHTS FOR
WEIGHT LOSS

The fast track to a slimmer, stronger, firmer body

SAM MURPHY

METRO BOOKS
NEW YORK

This 2006 edition published by Metro Books,
by arrangement with Kyle Cathie Limited

First published in Great Britain in 2006 by Kyle Cathie Limited as *Weights for Weight Loss*

Text © 2006 Sam Murphy
Photography © 2006 Guy Hearn
Additional photography: page 18 Stockbyte / Royalty Free / Getty Images, 144 Samboli / Alamy, 149 Dynamic Graphics Group / IT Stock Free / Alamy, 150 Dynamic Graphics Group / IT Stock Free / Alamy, 153 Jon Feingersh / Getty Images

Project editor: Caroline Taggart
Editorial assistant: Vicki Murrell
Copy editor: Sarah Epton
Designer: Rebecca Herriott
Illustrator: Peter Cox
Production: Sha Huxtable and Alice Holloway

Sam Murphy is hereby identified as the author of this work in accordance with Section 77 of the Copyright, Designs and Patents Act 1988.

Metro Books
122 Fifth Avenue
New York, NY 10011

ISBN-13: 978-0-7607-8188-3
ISBN-10: 0-7607-8188-5

Color separations by Colorscan
Printed and bound in Singapore by Tien-Wah Press

10 9 8 7 6 5 4 3 2

CONTENTS

INTRODUCTION

So you want to lose weight, shape up, and shed body fat? Then you need to be strong. I'm not talking about being strong enough to resist chocolate cake or a second helping of Sunday roast (although that inevitably helps!) – but about physical strength.

When we set our sights on weight loss, most of us turn to the kind of activities that get the heart pumping – like running, swimming, cycling, or aerobics classes. And while there is no doubt about the value of cardiovascular activity (for weight loss and general health), strength – or resistance – training is the unsung hero when it comes to maximizing daily energy expenditure and fat loss – and *really* streamlining your body shape.

But if you are serious about using weights for weight loss, that means dispensing with the ubiquitous can of baked beans as a makeshift dumbbell – many women squander their time in the gym by using weights that simply aren't challenging enough to trigger changes in the body. Others fail to benefit because they use poor technique or don't have any structure to their weights workout.

This book will show you how to incorporate strength training into your fitness regime (even if you don't yet have one!) in a safe, enjoyable, and above all *effective* way. You won't believe what a difference it will make to your weight loss efforts, your body shape, and size. But what's just as gratifying is the sense of empowerment you'll feel when you can lift a couple of heavy shopping bags (or kids) without a second thought…

Because there is no definitive 'strength training prescription' that gets the best results for every individual, *Using Your Weights for Weight Loss* will also help you to understand how your body type and shape is likely to respond to strength training, what other factors might influence the results you get and, most importantly, how to manipulate your workouts to maximize your own personal benefits.

There are a lot of myths and misconceptions about weight training out there but rest assured that you won't end up with big, bulging muscles, nor will you lose your aerobic fitness or flexibility. What you *will* lose is fat – revealing your new, firmer, more defined shape. You'll also reduce your risk of osteoporosis and back problems, stave off age-related declines in metabolism, muscle mass, and general function, maintain full range of motion in your joints and, perhaps most surprisingly of all, lower your risk of heart disease, high blood pressure, diabetes, and some cancers.

And all this can be achieved with just three strength-training workouts a week. You don't even need to go to a gym or pick up a dumbbell, as it's perfectly possible to train with alternative – or even no – equipment. The workouts in this book will show you how. You will also find the information you need to make smart eating choices so that you can lose body fat without starving yourself or feeling deprived and *keep* it off.

After all, anyone who tells you that you can successfully shed fat without addressing what you eat is stringing you along.

Using Your Weights for Weight Loss works because it is based on the sound scientific principles underpinning strength training, metabolism, and energy balance. No false promises. No complicated diet plans or baffling exercise regimes. Just a definitive weights workout that will reward you with a leaner, firmer, stronger body. Worth the weight…?

GIVE ME STRENGTH

What strength training is all about and why everyone should be doing it...

What exactly is strength? Put simply, it's the ability of a muscle to exert force and overcome resistance. That might not sound like something you are eager to devote your time to improving but there are a multitude of benefits to be gained from becoming stronger which go far beyond being able to shift heavy objects. How about looking leaner, improving muscle definition, getting a firmer, shapelier body, enhancing body composition, and boosting your calorie expenditure for starters? And there's more...

A few years back strength training didn't get much attention when people extolled the virtues of exercise. It was all about aerobic workouts. But there is now irrefutable evidence that strength training is not just desirable but *essential* for optimal health.

Getting the picture that it is well worth making strength training part of your life? Just in case you're not convinced, here are 12 compelling reasons – weight loss aside – to persuade you...

It helps your heart

If you think that the aerobic system isn't involved in resistance training, you are mistaken. For starters, it fuels recovery, not just between repetitions and sets of exercises but also following the session itself. It instigates heart-healthy changes in the cardiovascular system – such as allowing more blood to get to the muscle and enabling waste products to be cleared more efficiently. Of course, the heart itself is a muscle and strength training has been shown to increase the size of the heart chamber responsible for pumping blood around the body. This allows more blood to be delivered to the exercising muscles with every beat.

It lowers the risk of diabetes

Diabetes is one of the fastest increasing diseases in the Western world. Traditionally, aerobic exercise has been recommended to improve glucose metabolism but in a recent study four months of strength training increased glucose uptake by an average of 23% – indicating that it could be equally as effective. It also seems that strength training improves glucose metabolism both in subjects with normal glucose metabolism and those who already have an abnormal response. Researchers aren't exactly sure how it helps but recent studies suggest that resistance training increases the number and efficiency of glucose receptors in muscles so that the body doesn't need to produce as much insulin.

It reduces blood pressure

Strength training used to be thought to increase blood pressure but, increasingly, evidence shows that it can reduce blood pressure both acutely (as the result of a single session) and chronically (in the long term). This is especially good news because hypertension is associated with heart disease, stroke, and kidney problems. Improved strength also reduces stress on the heart. In a twelve-week study

subjects worked out with weights to strengthen the lower body muscles. By the end of the study period their blood pressure rose significantly less during lifting activities.

It bulks up your bones

Building bone density is the first line of defense against the debilitating disease osteoporosis that affects one in three women over the age of 50. Research shows that bone mineral density (BMD) is highly related to the strength of the muscles attached to those bones. In a research study, twice-weekly resistance training over the course of a year resulted in a 6.3% increase in bone mineral density of the lumbar spine. The surprising thing about this is that the women were post-menopausal – when bone density is usually plummeting. The control group in the study (who did no strength training) lost 3.7% of their bone density during that same year.

While weight bearing activities like running and high impact aerobics are great for bone density, they only influence the particular parts of the skeleton that are stressed a lot by the activity. As well as preserving bone density strength training reduces the risk of osteoporotic fractures, by improving balance and muscle strength, thereby reducing the risk of falls.

It preserves your joint health

Strength training isn't just good for muscles – it strengthens the connective tissues too – such as ligaments, tendons, and cartilage – while movement keeps the joint structures bathed in sticky synovial fluid. All these factors keep joints healthy and can even alleviate the symptoms of osteoarthritis.

It may improve your cholesterol profile

First, a quick cholesterol recap: HDL good, LDL bad! High levels of low density lipoprotein (LDL) and total cholesterol are associated with a higher risk of coronary heart disease, while high density lipoprotein (HDL) cholesterol is positively beneficial to heart health, helping to prevent the development of atherosclerosis. There's been conflicting evidence regarding whether strength training can help to improve cholesterol profile but it certainly seems that post-menopause (when heart-protective estrogen is out of the picture) resistance training can be very beneficial. In research from the University of Oklahoma post-menopausal women who took part in twelve weeks of resistance training using resistance bands, experienced a significant rise (13%) in HDL cholesterol levels despite the fact that they did not lose weight or body fat. The poorer the initial cholesterol profile the greater the subject's improvement.

It keeps you regular

Yup, strength training can improve your digestion! A study that involved thirteen weeks of strength training, including exercises for the abdominals, found a staggering 56% acceleration in gastrointestinal tract time (GITT). The reason this is desirable is because a long GITT is associated with colon cancer, not to mention digestive problems.

It's the way to an easier life

If you think strength training is all about aesthetics, think again. Put it this way: if you can lift a 20lb weight, that 10lb bag of shopping isn't going to pose a challenge. Being stronger helps you get through daily tasks with less effort and more energy. In fact, anyone reading this who has had children has already experienced the effects of 'progressive overload' strength training: first off when the baby was growing inside you and then after his or her birth, when you continued to nurse, pick up, and carry your little bundle of joy despite his or her rapidly advancing weight.

It can make you a better athlete

Even if your main fitness focus is an endurance activity such as running or cycling there is solid evidence that strength training can aid your performance. As well as making connective tissues more robust it also increases muscle power and makes movement patterns more efficient, so that you waste less energy. Being stronger will make you less injury-prone.

It makes you happier

Strength training can put a smile on your face! And the harder you work the happier you'll get, according to research from the Royal Prince Alfred Hospital in Sydney. Depressed adults were put on a high or low intensity-training strength program for eight weeks. At the end of the study period a reduction in depressive symptoms was directly associated with the amount of strength gained. Over half the high intensity group reported a 50% improvement. Sleep quality improved significantly in all the subjects too. But you need to keep it up: recent research found that as little as a week of no exercise resulted in an 85% drop in mood scores among regular gym rats!

It improves your body image

Strength training doesn't just improve your body, it also improves how you *feel* about your body. I can definitely attest to the feeling of empowerment you get when you can lift an Olympic bar in the gym when all the other girls are wielding 5lb dumbbells – or when you can place that six-pack of bottled water on the checkout without so much as a grunt!

It keeps you youthful

The average adult loses between $5^1/_2$ and 7 pounds of muscle mass every decade from around twenty years of age and experiences a 2–5% reduction in metabolic rate. As you'll find out in the next chapter, these two factors combine to form a potent fat-gaining force. But resistance training can prevent this. When you consider that muscle accounts for 16–22% of resting metabolic rate, it's easy to see how important it is not to let that muscle waste away.

So there you have it. But what about dropping excess pounds, shaping up, and losing body fat? The next section looks more closely at exactly how weight training works for weight loss.

HOW WEIGHTS WORK FOR WEIGHT LOSS

The lowdown on strength training and its effect on fat loss, energy expenditure, and body shape

So you want to lose weight. Surely you need to eat less and burn calories through exercise then? Absolutely. But if you are steering clear of weight training, believing that because it doesn't get you hot and sweaty it can't be much good for burning calories, then you are selling yourself short.

Strength training will help in three ways. It will burn calories, it will give you stronger muscles, which are more able to cope with the demands of weight-bearing aerobic exercise, and it will help you maintain your lean muscle mass as you decrease calorie intake so you don't lose precious metabolically active muscle tissue. The single biggest contributor in determining your total daily energy (calorie) expenditure is your resting metabolic rate (or RMR – the amount of energy your body expends just keeping itself going on a typical day). A low RMR is an independent predictor of future weight gain but the single most important factor in *determining* your RMR is the amount of lean muscle tissue you have in your body – which is why weight loss experts now recommend combining aerobic exercise and strength training with diet to produce successful results.

Another important benefit of strength training is that it will allow you to *enjoy* becoming more active. Being overweight is not an impediment to successful strength training and in fact, brand new research on young people found that it was actually the most overweight kids who fared best in the gym. Strength training is a great first step to becoming more active and healthy as there's no bouncing about, no excessive stress on joints, and no need to feel self-conscious. Whether you do it at home alone, or in a busy gym, strength training is a very individual pursuit that you can tackle with dignity and focus. Let's look at how it works for weight loss…

The high cost of strength training

Exercise at any intensity – whether it's walking, running, weight lifting, or circuit training – burns calories and utilizes fat. The number of calories and the proportion of fat is what varies – but while lower-intensity exercise burns a higher proportion of fat, higher-intensity exercise burns more calories overall – and weight training can certainly be considered to be a high-intensity activity (when done properly, of course).

But it isn't just the calorie 'cost' of the sessions themselves that make weight training such a crucial part of the weight loss equation. Studies suggest that resistance training has an effect on average daily metabolic rate and energy expenditure through other means too. In an eighteen-week intervention study from the University of Limburg in Holland, average daily metabolic rate increased by 9.5% and energy expenditure by 10% as a result of twice-weekly training. Less than half of this increase could be attributed to the calorie cost of the workouts themselves, so positive effects on metabolism must explain the rest.

What are you made of?

There are two important factors at work. Firstly, research shows that by increasing your 'fat-free mass' (the proportion of your body weight made up of anything other than fat), your body burns more calories on a daily basis. Therefore, altering your body composition to include less fat and more muscle is a good thing for weight loss (not to mention heart health). At the very least, resistance training causes a short term hike in resting metabolic rate.

Secondly, all exercise has an 'afterburn' effect, known as 'excess post-exercise oxygen consumption' (EPOC) – a period during which additional energy is needed to help the body replenish depleted fuel stores following a workout. This recovery period following exercise is almost entirely fueled by fat oxidation (oxidation just means burning or 'use'). The intensity of the exercise and length of the session dictates the amount of energy used – the greater the intensity the better. Research has shown that fat oxidation can last up to three hours post resistance exercise and burns a significant number of extra calories.

Lose the fat, keep the muscle

The case for weight training becomes even stronger when you bring reduced calorie intake into the equation. When you cut calories, more than a quarter of the pounds you lose aren't fat – they consist of water, muscle tissue, and even bone. Now, the relevance of this is that muscle is a demanding type of tissue – it needs to be fed calories constantly to keep it functioning.

The more muscle you have, the more calories you burn whether you are walking along the street or doing barbell squats. Fat, in contrast, is quite happy to just sit there without making any demands for energy.

A study, from the University of Texas, Austin, looked at the effects of twelve weeks of either high-intensity endurance or resistance training on resting metabolic rate in men aged 18–35. After training both exercise groups showed significant declines in body fat. Resting metabolic rate did not significantly change after either training regime but there *was* a definite increase in energy expenditure. These results suggest that both endurance and resistance training may help prevent the attenuation of RMR normally seen during dieting.

STRONG WORDS

WHY NOT JUST DIET?

Calorie restriction has been shown to have a very positive effect on weight loss in the short term. But, in a study review looking at research on calorie cutting and weight loss over 25 years, it was found that the average person regained 35% of the weight they'd lost within a year. Diets that restrict calories to 1200 or below can reduce metabolic rate by as much as 20%. It's also been shown that exercise causes 'protein sparing' (literally, your body tries to hold on to its protein stores), which helps to maintain muscle mass.

And finally…

There's yet another reason why strength training is such a string to your weight loss bow. It has a remarkable effect on the shape and outline of your body. Fat is like a big sponge while muscle is dense, like stone. A pound of fat takes up as much as five times more space than a pound of muscle which is why you'll look so much trimmer after strength training.

And here's the scientific evidence on six ways weights work for weight loss…

A flatter tummy

In a study in the journal *Medicine & Science in Sports & Exercise* strength training three times a week, using two sets of each exercise, reduced levels of fat both under the skin on the abdomen and in between the organs in the abdominal region. In all, the female subjects lost 3³/₄lb of pure fat in 25 weeks.

Reduced body fat

In research published in the *Journal of Strength and Conditioning Research* women over 30 were assigned to a twelve-week weight-training program, working out three days a week. Both body fat and skinfold girths (measurements of the amount of skin that can be 'pinched' at specific body sites) were lower, while fat-free mass increased.

Better body composition

In a study published in the *Journal of the American Dietetic Association*, the effect of weight training on resting metabolic rate, fat-free mass, strength, and dietary intake was expenditure increasing by over 220 calories per day. RMR also increased by 6.8%. Even after adjusting the figures for the calorie cost of the training sessions themselves total daily energy expenditure was *still* significantly higher, meaning that both RMR and increased physical activity contributed to the higher figure.

Higher fat-free mass

A Japanese study found that fat-free mass and the amount of high-intensity physical activity performed were the strongest determinants of total daily energy expenditure, accounting for 51% of it.

Greater afterburn

A study in *Medicine & Science in Sport & Exercise* found that 45 minutes of resistance training elevated metabolism for two hours afterwards, resulting in an additional expenditure of 155 calories.

assessed for twelve weeks in young women. The women showed a significant increase in fat-free mass of $4^1/_2$lb, a highly respectable decrease in body fat percentage of 2.6% and significant increases in strength. RMR did not change significantly and neither did body weight. So, in this case, it seems that weight training had a beneficial effect on body composition.

Higher total energy expenditure

In a study from the University of Alabama that looked at older adults, 26 weeks of resistance training resulted in total daily energy

Hopefully, you are now convinced that weight training is something you simply can't leave out of your weight loss strategy. But stop right there! Before you skim over this section in your keenness to get on with the *Using Your Weights for Weight Loss* program, I think it is important to understand a little about what muscles are and how they work. I'm not asking you to sign up for a physiology course but the whistle-stop tour in the next section will help you learn how to get the most out of resistance training and make you understand why doing biceps curls with a can of baked beans in each hand is, frankly, a waste of time.

BONING UP ON MUSCLES

Are you sitting comfortably? Then I'll begin...

What is muscle?

At the most basic level, muscle is simply the tissue in the body that initiates movement. That's not to say it does such a remarkable thing all on its own (the cardiovascular, nervous and hormonal systems are all involved) – but muscle is what actually enables us to move, by contracting and pulling on bones. There are more than 430 skeletal muscles in the body and virtually every move we make involves the action of more than one of them.

A closer look

Let's take a muscle, say, the biceps muscle in the arm (the one Popeye is always flexing), and have a closer look. A muscle is made up of thousands of long thin fibers (the term muscle fiber and muscle cell are used interchangeably) – about the diameter of a human hair. Each individual fiber is surrounded by connective tissue and groups of fibers are arranged into bundles (consisting of up to 150 fibers each), also encased in connective tissue. Then the whole muscle is

The make-up of a muscle

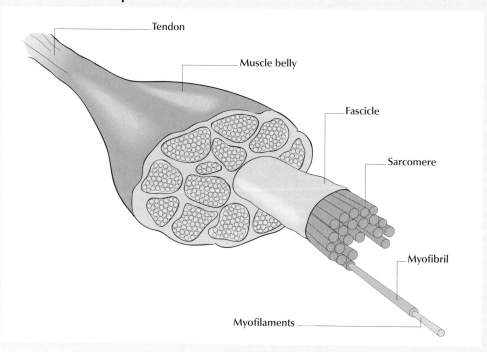

Tendon

Muscle belly

Fascicle

Sarcomere

Myofibril

Myofilaments

sheathed in yet another layer of connective tissue – the epimysium. All these layers of connective tissue join up to the tendon – which is what makes the structure so robust – and it is via these tendons that muscles pull on bone. To cause movement, each end of the muscle is attached to a different bone – one end is called the insertion, the other end the origin. So, for example, the biceps muscle is attached at one end to the radius (a bone in the forearm) and at the other end to the scapula or shoulder blade. When the biceps contracts the forearm moves towards the shoulder, as in a biceps curl.

The muscle fiber is divided into a series of blocks called sarcomeres. As far as muscle contraction is concerned the most important components of each sarcomere are the myofibrils (basically, these are strands of two proteins, called actin and myosin, which are arranged in bundles lengthways along the muscle fiber). These myofibrils are the key structures responsible for facilitating muscle contraction – since it is the action of one locking on to the other that draws the sarcomeres closer together, shortening the muscle and pulling on the tendon… and the bone… and causing movement.

How does muscle get stronger?

Muscle will only be as strong as it needs to be. If you rarely lift a finger, let alone a dumbbell, then your muscles will have adapted to cope with this low level of demand and, consequently, will find more taxing activities (like getting up out of a chair)

a challenge. To make a muscle stronger you need to 'overload' it. That is, you need to put it under more stress than it is accustomed to. Now, correct me if I'm wrong, but I wouldn't have thought getting a can of baked beans out the cupboard causes you to buckle under the weight… So neither is it (nor a 2lb hand weight or a bottle of mineral water) sufficient to create overload or instigate the adaptations needed to make your muscles stronger.

A muscle's 'pulling power' is dependent on the number of actin-myosin bonds (those protein strands) per myofibril. If you want to pull harder, you need more of 'em. So how do you get them? Tiny amounts of damage, caused by training, initiate the creation of further strands being added to the myofibril, and, indeed, more myofibrils being added to the fiber. More myofibrils mean the fiber gets physically bigger, as it has more 'bundles' packed along its length. And the increased thickness of the muscle fiber gives it a greater ability to develop force.

It is worth knowing that while you can make the fibers *bigger*, it is not believed that you can change the *number* of fibers within a muscle – that is determined by your genetics.

Hitting a nerve

The second thing that changes in order to increase strength relates to the communication between the central nervous system and the muscles (the neuromuscular system). A special type of nerve cell, called a motor neuron, acts as the 'governor' to a specific group of fibers (which could be anything from several hundred to just a handful) and it is this that gives the signal to contract. Muscles that have to do very precise actions may have just one fiber per motor neuron but bigger muscles with less particular jobs will have several hundred fibers being served by one motor neuron. A motor neuron and the muscle fibers it activates are collectively called a motor unit. When the motor neuron receives a message from the central nervous system (ground control) saying 'Move!,' it, in turn, tells all its muscle fibers to contract.

The motor neuron makes all the fibers within the motor unit contract and develop force at the same time… But don't think that each *muscle* consists of just one motor unit – in fact, a muscle consists of *scores* of motor units and they don't all contribute to every movement. The number that is recruited is proportional to the force needed to initiate the movement – the greater the force, the more motor units recruited.

If you were to try to lift an iron bar, for example, most of the motor units in the biceps would be recruited, whereas if it were just a cup of tea only a small number would get involved. Whatever the movement the motor units involved are not continually active. Instead, they switch on and off at different times but they do this so fast that you get a smooth contraction (think of a wave).

All systems go

The question of how many motor units will be fired at any one time is determined by your training experience and efficiency, not to mention your genes. At first, the mechanism is very crude – and the nervous system tends to underestimate how many 'workers' it needs for the job. But, as you train regularly, you become more effective and fire up more motor units every time, so you get more 'hands on deck' and, consequently, greater strength. In strength training newbies, strength gains over the first few weeks of training are mostly to do with improved neuromuscular pathways rather than physiological changes in the muscle – which set in later. That's why you can't expect to see an increase in muscle size (known as hypertrophy) in the first couple of months. But, however much you train, you cannot change the number of fibers per motor unit. This varies between individuals and is one of the reasons why some people can achieve greater muscle size and strength far more easily than others.

But whether it is just a couple of motor units or a few hundred that take part, the order in which they are recruited is always the same. This 'sequential order' is related to the type of muscle fiber that the motor unit

contains. Yup! There ain't just one type of fiber to get your head around...

Fiber types

Fibers are broadly divided into type 1 and type 2 – and the distinction relates to whether the fiber develops force slowly or rapidly. We all have some of both but the type that predominates varies from person to person and muscle to muscle and this will influence – to some extent – the kind of activity you are best suited to. Postural muscles, such as the soleus in the calf, have a high percentage of slow-twitch fibers, to allow them to provide stability; while dynamic muscles, such as the quads in the front of the thigh, have a mixture of fast- and slow-twitch fibers, to allow them to execute both low-intensity (such as walking) and high-intensity (like jumping) activities. Endurance athletes tend to have a lot of type 1, or slow-twitch fibers. (Muscle biopsies have revealed as much as 99% slow-twitch fibers in the calf muscles of marathon runners.) These fibers are highly resistant to fatigue due to their ability to process lots of oxygen but they tend to be recruited mainly at low intensities of effort (such as picking up that cup of tea). Type 2 or fast-twitch fibers, on the other hand, are associated with muscle power, strength, and speed – and only kick in when the intensity of the effort required increases.

The major muscles

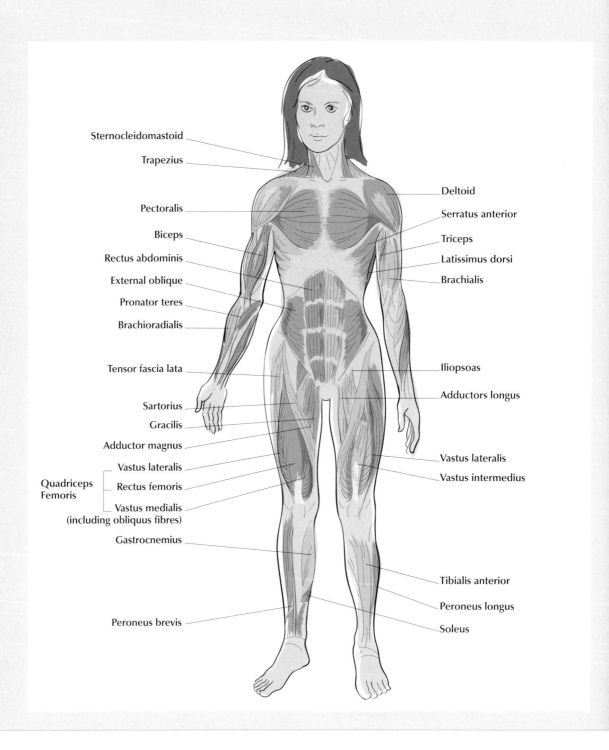

Sternocleidomastoid

Trapezius

Pectoralis

Biceps

Rectus abdominis

External oblique

Pronator teres

Brachioradialis

Tensor fascia lata

Sartorius

Gracilis

Adductor magnus

Quadriceps Femoris
- Vastus lateralis
- Rectus femoris
- Vastus medialis (including obliquus fibres)

Gastrocnemius

Peroneus brevis

Deltoid

Serratus anterior

Triceps

Latissimus dorsi

Brachialis

Iliopsoas

Adductors longus

Vastus lateralis

Vastus intermedius

Tibialis anterior

Peroneus longus

Soleus

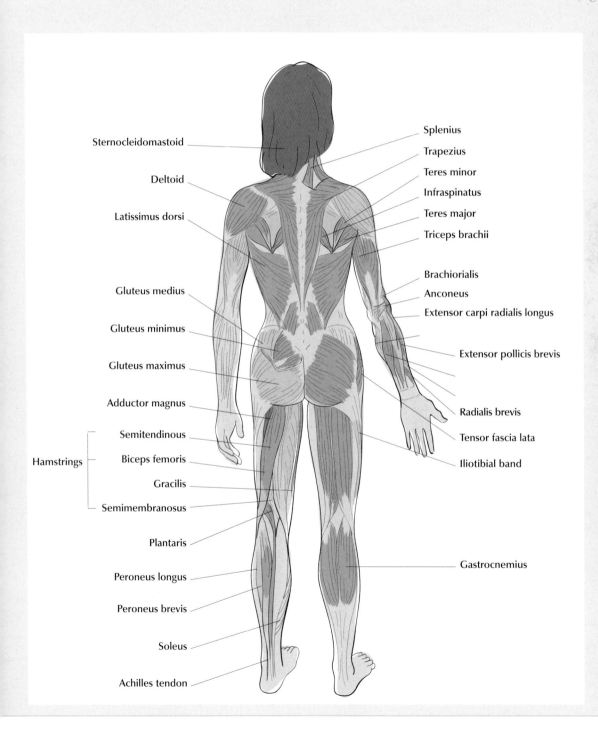

Sternocleidomastoid

Deltoid

Latissimus dorsi

Gluteus medius

Gluteus minimus

Gluteus maximus

Adductor magnus

Hamstrings

Semitendinous

Biceps femoris

Gracilis

Semimembranosus

Plantaris

Peroneus longus

Peroneus brevis

Soleus

Achilles tendon

Splenius

Trapezius

Teres minor

Infraspinatus

Teres major

Triceps brachii

Brachiorialis

Anconeus

Extensor carpi radialis longus

Extensor pollicis brevis

Radialis brevis

Tensor fascia lata

Iliotibial band

Gastrocnemius

What it all means

And here's the important bit, as far as strength training is concerned. (At last!) Since the motor units are recruited in sequential order, from slow twitch to fast twitch, it follows that the only way to train a muscle in its entirety (getting the maximum number of motor units involved) is to expose it to high – and increasingly challenging – loads to ensure they all get 'a piece of the action.' That is why doing lots of reps with a light weight won't build strength or size. No muscle fiber – fast or slow twitch – is overloaded. In a nutshell, light weights don't present enough load to change the physiology of any fiber.

Makes sense? Well, just to confuse things, there are two types of type 2 fibers – known as type 2a and type 2b. While 2b are the true power rangers, the type 2a fibers sit on the fence and, depending on the type of training you do, can be made to act either more like endurance-based type 1 or power-based type 2b fibers. In other words, they can be trained for stamina or strength. This is very important when it comes to program planning, as you can't have your cake and eat it – at least, not within one particular muscle. That's why knowing the basics of muscle physiology is so useful, when you want to train for real results.

Why stronger doesn't mean bigger

There is probably one question that you are still asking by this point. Is it possible to get firmer and stronger, without getting bigger muscles? The answer is yes. If you were to look at a muscle in cross-section, you'd see that there is space between those bundles of long thin fibers. In an untrained muscle, there is lots of space. When you train, the fibers get bigger. But that doesn't mean the muscle *itself* gets bigger, as the muscle fibers simply take up more of the free space in the muscle by becoming more tightly packed. This – along with a host of other physiological adaptations – is why muscles 'firm up' when you train them. And no amount of reps with those baked bean cans is going to get you there. This will not actually instigate the adaptations that allow the fibers to get thicker, so will achieve neither definition nor firmness.

If you don't want to increase the overall size of the muscle you can stop increasing the overload, once the muscle has gained sufficient strength and firmness, to maintain this new level of 'tone' (see right) without adding volume. Continue to 'overload' the muscle, though, and it will increase slightly in diameter, as the fibers and myofibrils thicken.

The results

So now we know a little about how muscles function, let's look at how to train them to get the results we want. How strength training affects you as an individual depends on a number of factors – most importantly, arguably, the way you train (in terms of frequency, weight, number of reps and sets) but also your genes, gender, age, what other physical activity you do, your diet, and even your technique. The next chapter will help you gain an idea of how your body is likely to respond.

STRONG WORDS

CAN YOU JUST 'TONE UP'?

We all use the word 'tone' as though it is a specific training goal but, really, all tone means is 'a state of slight tension' – in other words, the muscle is slightly active, rather than totally passive. If muscles are accustomed to being active they tend to have a higher level of tone than in people who are inactive and don't use their muscles much. Tone is related to shape, or definition, in a muscle because when a muscle contracts it shortens and bulges as the fibers overlap one another, giving more shape. So, yes, strength training will improve your muscle tone. However, definition – or lack of it – is very often more to do with too much body fat covering the muscle rather than a lack of muscle shape. It may also be due to poor flexibility. Pat Fox, strength and conditioning specialist at South Bank University, points out that working through a full range of motion, and practicing flexibility work, are essential to achieve a streamlined non-bulky look.

HOW WILL WEIGHTS WORK FOR ME?

The factors that affect the results you are likely to get from strength training and how to get the best results for you

This may come as some surprise to you but even if you and your best friend do exactly the same workout, with the same amount of weight, the same number of times a week, there is no guarantee that you will get the same results.

Lots of factors affect how your body responds to weights. Gender is probably the biggest factor because of the huge differences in levels of testosterone and other anabolic (muscle building) hormones in men and women; but women's natural testosterone levels can also vary from person to person. Your age, training status, body shape and size, predominant type of muscle fibers, diet, and good old DNA will all also have an influence on the results you can achieve.

Two scientists, Paul Thompson and Eric Hoffman, demonstrated the wild variation in response to working with weights by recruiting 700 male and 700 female newbies to lift weights for twelve weeks. The biceps and triceps muscles of the subjects were scanned using magnetic resonance imaging (MRI) to precisely measure muscle size, while special machines were used to assess strength in each of these muscles at the start of the study. At the end of the study, during which time these muscles were trained intensively, some subjects had built size but not strength. Others had built considerable strength but not size. Still others had gained both and a handful didn't seem to have got either stronger or bigger, proving that there is undoubtedly a genetic component involved in how your body will respond to weights. (That's not to say you can't influence the way your body responds by manipulating some of the training variables – but we'll come on to that later.) First let's look at factors specific to the fairer sex…

How being a dame affects the results

On average, a woman has around 50–60% of the absolute strength of a man in the upper body and about 70% of the lower body strength. Women tend to be smaller, shorter, and lighter – and carry more body fat – than men. Even when you factor in the smaller body size, the higher level of body fat remains, because women have a supply of 'essential' fat to cope with the demands of pregnancy and lactation. So overall, a woman's body composition is geared toward more fat and less muscle than a man's. On average, skeletal muscle accounts for about 38% of total body weight in men and 31% in women.

STRONG WORDS

GIRTH CONTROL

In studies looking at the effect of weight training on women the greatest increase in various body girths, as a result of between twelve and twenty weeks of training, was 0.4–0.6cm, proving that strength workouts are hardly going to give you strapping shoulders and bulging calves. A quite considerable *decrease* in body girths where fat tends to be stored, such as the hips, thighs and abdomen, is commonly found. In one twelve-week study, tummy girth decreased by 0.2–1.1cm, while a ten-week program resulted in hip, thigh and abdominal circumferences decreasing by 0.2–0.7cm.

We girls also tend to have a smaller hip to shoulder ratio, a wider pelvis and a greater 'Q' angle; the angle at which the thighbone travels from the hip to the knee. With smaller muscle fibers – and a tenth of the muscle-building hormone testosterone that a man has – women aren't primed for building big, bulky muscles. But they absolutely *can* get stronger, firmer, and shapelier – and tip the body composition balance towards less fat and more muscle through working with weights.

The average woman can expect to see a strength improvement of 25–30% within six months of starting a resistance training program.

Confession time

Despite the title of this book, I have to admit that resistance training may not help you shed body weight. Disappointed? Well, consider this – would you rather fit your 130lb frame into size 14 jeans, or your 140lb frame into a size 10? The truth is, muscle weighs a lot more than fat (a third again as much, in fact) but I promise you will look and feel trimmer and slimmer by altering your body composition to consist of more muscle and less fat, regardless of whether you lose weight. You *will* see a change in your body silhouette and you *will* see shape and tone. That goes for whether you are a classic pear-shaped woman, an apple, a stick insect, or an hourglass. Happily, there is no physiological reason that any body type cannot increase muscle mass and decrease fat mass and gain better body definition. But, of course, you can't actually change the basic structure of your body – think of it as the 'blank canvas' you have to work with…

What's your type?

Scientists refer to your body shape as your somatotype. William Sheldon's somatotyping system, developed in the 1950s, is still widely used though it has been rather oversimplified.

Sheldon talked in terms of the relative dominance of certain body characteristics when he defined his three somatotypes. Endomorphy referred to roundness, mesomorphy referred to muscularity, and ectomorphy referred to linearity. He used a scale of 1–7 for each type to give an overall score. So, for example, a score of 1-7-1 would indicate an extremely mesomorphic person. Nowadays, people use the system to brand one person as an 'ectomorph,' another as an 'endomorph.' But, if it were really that simple, wouldn't an endomorph who lost lots of weight become an ectomorph? Body typing is only useful if it reflects body qualities that cannot be changed, such as the ratio of your shoulder-to-hip width or the length of your bones.

Sheldon's somatotyping is not the only method used to classify body types: another system refers to glandular dominances, in which the 'thyroid' type replaces the ectomorph, the 'adrenal' type replaces the mesomorph and the 'pituitary' type replaces the endomorph. This body typing system introduces a fourth category for women only, termed 'gonadal,' which is associated with the stereotypical 'pear-shaped' female – narrow shoulders and wide hips. Regardless of the system used few of us represent textbook versions of one particular somatotype – but we do tend to have more features from one type than another.

Here are some of the classic characteristics associated with each type of dominance…

Endomorphs – Pear shaped – shoulders that are narrower relative to hips – rounded, soft. Short limbs, long torso. Short musculature. If you circle your wrist with your opposite thumb and middle finger and the digits don't meet you may be endomorphic. Picture a trapezius.

Mesomorphs – broad shouldered, thick chested, narrow waisted and muscular with a long torso. Usually well proportioned. Triangular shaped body (wider shoulders than hips). Finds it easy to build muscle mass. If you circle your wrist with your opposite thumb and middle finger and the digits just touch it indicates a dominance of mesomorphy. Visualize an upside down trapezius.

Ectomorphs – short upper body, long arms and legs, long narrow feet and hands and very little fat storage. This body type has a narrow chest and narrow shoulders and long, thin muscles; quite 'straight up and down' (not much of a waist). Narrow bones – if you circle your wrist with your opposite thumb and middle finger and

the digits overlap you are most likely an ectomorph. Visualize a rectangle.

How does your body type affect your training?

It's all very well knowing that you are, say, mainly mesomorphic but what does it mean when it comes to training? After all, it's only worth knowing if it has some influence on what you should actually do. A lot of nonsense is written about this – such as if you are endomorphic you should concentrate on aerobic exercise while if you are ectomorphic you should do less aerobic exercise and more weights. This kind of advice totally disregards the issue of heart health and the importance of a balanced program and implies that you can't be a slim endomorph or an overweight ectomorph, which simply isn't the case.

A classic illustration of this is the notion that it is 'difficult' for a pear-shaped endomorph to gain muscle, especially in the lower body. In fact a larger frame – whether it be at the hips or shoulders – indicates a *greater* potential for muscular development, as the surface area of the muscle needs to be larger to span the greater distance from origin to insertion.

Since body fat storage predominates around the pelvic frame, however – whether that be around the abdominal region or the hips, buttocks, and thighs – a wider pelvic girdle gives greater potential for fat storage too, which explains the tendency for an endomorphic body shape to have a high propensity for body fat storage.

Working from the inside out

The factors we've discussed so far are beyond your control – such as your sex, body type, and limb length. Another major reason that people don't get the results they expect from strength training is that they inevitably take their own postural idiosyncrasies, muscle imbalances, weaknesses, and tightnesses with them into the gym. In other words, few – if any – of us are starting off with a truly blank canvas.

Say, for example, you start doing lots of chest exercises to strengthen and tone your pectorals but already have a rounded shoulder posture. Without the inclusion of flexibility work for the pecs, and strengthening of the opposing muscle groups in the back, you will simply exacerbate the existing postural problem. Or you begin doing squats with tight hip flexors and poor knee mechanics and end up with a sore back and knee pain.

While I am not claiming that you can reverse the maladaptions of a couple of decades in a matter of weeks, it is still a wise idea to spend a little time on improving posture and redressing imbalances before you even pick up a weight – which is why the *Using Your Weights for Weight Loss* program begins with the Foundation Workout on page 58. It does exactly what it says – it lays the foundation for you to become stronger without reinforcing poor postural and movement habits, enabling you to develop long, lean, and balanced muscles that work efficiently and are injury-resistant. Even if you feel you are in good shape I still recommend that you follow the Foundation Workout for two to three weeks before moving on to the more demanding programs. See 'Three easy steps to better body awareness', opposite, to get you off on the right foot. You can start practicing these moves RIGHT NOW!

STRONG WORDS

LONG LIMBS, LONG MUSCLES

When it comes to relative strength, shorter-limbed people have an advantage over the lankier-limbed, because the latter have to exert a force over a longer distance. (For example, in a bench press the bar has to travel further until the arms are straight.) It's also harder for the longer-limbed to gain definition and shape, as the muscle itself (which, you'll remember, attaches at both ends to bone) is physically longer and therefore more spread out. But in most cases, this is the exact long, lean look many women want to achieve.

Three easy steps to better body awareness

Mastering these three techniques will put you on track to better posture and body awareness ensuring you get the most out of every move in the *Weights for Weight Loss* Workout. It will also minimize your risk of injury, both during exercise and in normal daily activities.

The trunk muscles

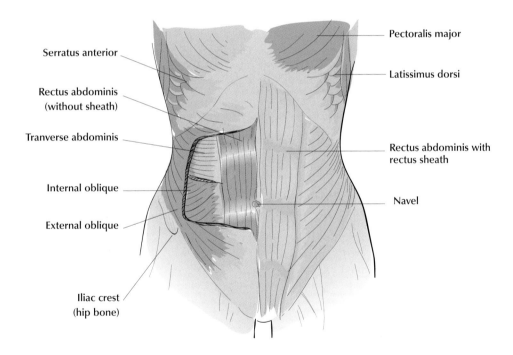

Serratus anterior

Rectus abdominis
(without sheath)

Tranverse abdominis

Internal oblique

External oblique

Iliac crest
(hip bone)

Pectoralis major

Latissimus dorsi

Rectus abdominis with
rectus sheath

Navel

Engaging the core

Engaging the core is really just a posh way of saying 'pull your tummy in.' But you have to learn how to identify and 'engage' or 'switch on' the right muscles. These are the deep muscles of the back, waist, and abdominals – known collectively as the 'core' muscles (see illustration on previous page) – whose role it is to protect and support the spine and provide a solid base for movement. Engaging the core muscles is fundamental to good posture, stability, a flatter abdomen, and more efficient movement.

1 To get a feel of the muscles you are trying to get to (as they lie deep below the surface of the tummy) kneel, sit, or stand and place your fingertips 2 inches in and 1 inch down from your hipbones and feign a cough – you should feel the muscles contract involuntarily under your fingertips. Got it?

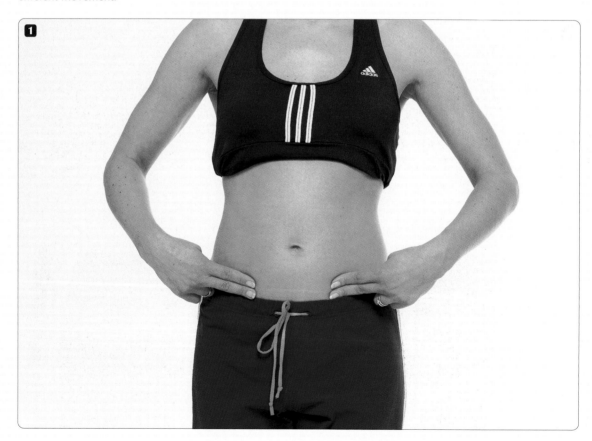

2 Now inhale and, as you exhale, start pulling up the pelvic floor (as if you were trying to stop yourself from peeing). This works because the lower fibers of the deep-set transversus abdominis muscle actually intermingle with the pelvic floor muscles. Continue to pull in and up, using those muscles you located in the cough, imagining you are doing up a zip fastener from your pubic bone to your navel.

3 It may help to take one hand to your lower back (palm away) and the other to your tummy (palm touching). You should feel the tummy pull away from the front hand but you don't want to feel the back pushing into the hand behind you. The spine remains still as the core engages but don't hold your breath. Build up to progressively longer holds and practice regularly throughout the day.

Setting the shoulder blades (scapulae)

Setting the shoulder blades makes your upper body more stable, injury resistant, and ensures that bigger, stronger muscles don't take over the job of the smaller ones and cause imbalances. Draw the shoulder blades back and slightly down, anchoring them at the top of the back of the ribcage. You should feel the chest lift and open slightly. A good way of getting the feeling is to hold a resistance tube in each hand behind your back and gently draw the hands away from each other until you feel a tension in the middle of the upper back. That is how the shoulder blades should feel when they are 'set.'

Standing tall

Stand with feet below your hipbones. Ensure the weight is evenly distributed between the front and back of the feet and between the left and right feet. Pull up through the arches of the feet and ensure all toes have contact with the ground. Pull up through the legs and ensure your buttocks have some tension in them but aren't clenched. Keep the hips square and level. Lengthen through the spine and engage the core, imaging the torso 'growing' out of the pelvis. Drop the rib cage, drawing the lower ribs down towards the pubic bone. Relax the shoulders, draw the spine deep into the back and gently open the chest and front of the shoulders by turning your thumbs to face the front (your little finger should be parallel to your trouser seam). Keep the neck long, the chin slightly retracted, and allow the head to sit squarely on top of the spine. Breathe freely.

Whether you are going to follow any of the programs in this book, or intend to create your own workout with the knowledge you've gained – it is important to follow the 'rules' of training and know a little about strength training terminology and protocols. You'll find all you need to know in the next chapter.

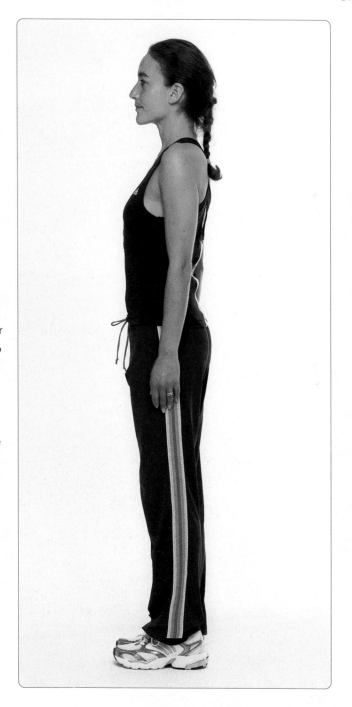

THE RULES

Follow the rules to ensure you train safely and effectively
– and get the results you want.

Can there *really* be a whole section on how to lift weights? Surely lifting and lowering a dumbbell can't be that complex! Well no, not once you know the ground rules. But even once you have got to grips with these, it doesn't mean they are set in stone. As you have probably guessed by now, there is no set, definitive formula for strength training that works for all goals and all people.

Crack an egg and you can make an omelet or a meringue, you can scramble it, poach, fry, or boil it. It's how you cook it, what you add and what kind of utensils you use to cook it that makes it turn out one way or another. And it's exactly the same with strength training!

There's an acronym that strength and conditioning specialists use, known as the 'SAID' principle. It stands for 'specific adaptation to imposed demands' and what it means is that the type of demand you place on your body dictates the type of changes that will occur. As a simple example, if you took up running, putting in four sessions of 45 minutes a week, your body would respond very differently from if you took up yoga – or weight training. The SAID principle also holds true *within* strength training. For example, lots of reps with a light weight and brief rests will have a very different outcome from short, heavy sets with long rests, as we will find out in just a moment.

Getting with the program

The American College of Sports Medicine's resistance training guidelines include the following advice (don't worry if you don't understand some of the terminology used – it is all explained over the following pages):

- Use both concentric and eccentric muscle actions.

- Use both single- and multiple-joint exercises (isolated and compound moves).

- Order exercises to optimize the quality of the workout (by training large before small muscle groups, doing multiple-joint exercises before single-joint exercises and higher-intensity before lower-intensity exercises).

- Beginners training for strength should use a weight corresponding to their 8–12 repetition maximum (RM).

- For intermediate to advanced strength training, use a wider loading range i.e. instead of just doing between 8–12 reps you can do between 1–12, experimenting with heavier weights with fewer reps.

- When you can comfortably perform 1 or 2 more repetitions than the number you set yourself, increase the weight by 2–10%.

- The recommendation for training frequency is 2–3 days a week for novice and intermediate training and 4–5 days a week for advanced training.

STRONG WORDS

A MOVING TALE

Muscle contractions are divided into three main types. An *isometric* contraction is when the muscle is producing a force but not changing in length. A perfect example of this is core stability work, such as the navel to spine hold on page 64 – you are holding the core stabilizers firm, while other parts of the body move.

Isometric contractions will strengthen muscles but only in and around the position in which the contraction is held. For example, if you did that exercise where you 'sit' with your back against a wall with your knees bent at a right angle, you'd only see increased strength in the thigh muscles at 90 degrees and perhaps 20 degrees either side of that.

In strength training you commonly have muscle contractions where the muscle first shortens and then lengthens as it exerts force, known as isotonic actions. For example, when your biceps contract to bend your arm the muscle shortens. This is called a *concentric action*. And then, when you lower the arm back down, the biceps have to control the descent of the arm – the contraction is happening while the muscle lengthens. This is called an *eccentric* action.

- Higher-volume, multiple-set programs are recommended for maximizing hypertrophy, with loads corresponding to 1–12 RM, with emphasis on the 6–12 RM zone using 1– to 2-minute rest periods between sets performed at a moderate speed.

- For local muscular endurance training, it is recommended that light to moderate loads (40–60% of 1 RM) be performed for high repetitions using short rest periods.

- All strength training should use the principle of periodization, in which a planned training program is divided into phases, each of which has a specific purpose or focus.

The ACSM points out that their guidelines need to be considered within the context of individual needs. It's also worth bearing in mind that even if you did find the 'perfect' formula – it wouldn't last long because, if there is one crucial ingredient to a successful strength training program, it is variety that stops both you and your muscles from getting bored!

That's progress

Another crucial element is remembering that, as you get stronger, you need to increase what's known as the 'training load.' It sounds obvious but I am always amazed by the number of people who get stuck in a rut with those 1lb biceps curls or twenty crunches. Once your body becomes comfortable with the workout you are presenting it you need to increase the challenge. Otherwise, you will fail to continue making improvements. This is known as 'progressive overload'. Now, increasing the training load can be achieved in a number of ways. The most obvious one is to increase the weight but you can also increase the number of reps or sets, or the frequency with which you exercise that muscle group. Note that word 'progressive' however – it means that you should increase the training load by a small amount – not pile it on all at once!

What are my strength training options?

As I promised in the introduction, you don't need to be a gym member to get into strength training. You can work with any type of resistance – including your own body weight (when working against gravity), elastic tubing, dumbbells, barbells, medicine balls – or, of course, the weight-training machines designed to train each muscle group. All have their place in a balanced program and practicalities – such as space, availability, convenience, or cost – may dictate what you choose to work with but the gold standard is generally considered to be free weights.

Free vs fixed weights

A free weight is one that isn't attached to anything, such as a dumbbell or barbell, while a 'fixed' weight moves in the plane and range dictated by the machine it is attached to. Because you aren't supported by anything as you exercise with free weights they demand greater effort and recruit more muscles in order to stabilize other joints while the movement is taking place. They also mimic real life more than fixed machines. After all, when you get a heavy box off a high shelf there isn't a machine providing stability and support for you…. Also, training with free weights burns more calories – as you engage more muscles in order to stabilize the body and assist the movement – not to mention having to lift and carry the weights around.

So what's the benefit of machines? Well, there are some movements that it is difficult to perform without the help of a machine (the lat pulldown is a good example) – and, of course, variety is the spice of life.

Traditionally, resistance training machines are recommended to beginners for ease of use and safety. Granted, you are less likely to clunk yourself on the head if you use the triceps pushdown machine rather than do a supine French press, for example. And you are also far less able to do the exercise 'wrong,' as the direction and range of motion is controlled and limited by the machine. But many experts now argue that this isn't necessarily a good thing and believe that using a combination of free weights, body weight, and stability balls better teaches people to stabilize themselves and control their range of motion. Also, since machines are designed to fit 'Mr Average,' they won't always fit you – although the array of adjustments that can be made to help you 'fit' better into a machine is impressive on today's hi-tech machinery.

At the end of the day, it's your choice. Research in the journal *Medicine & Science in Sport & Exercise* found no significant difference in strength gains in a free-weight bench press compared to a chest press machine so, if you like the familiarity of the machines, you aren't selling yourself short in strength terms. Weights machines can also help build confidence and are less intimidating for newcomers than the free weights area in a gym.

Exercise balls, medicine balls, and resistance tubing

Exercise balls or Swiss balls (basically, overgrown Spacehoppers with no ears) have become ubiquitous in gyms these days, and for good reason. Any exercise you do on the ball will be more challenging than it is on a stable surface. As well as coping with the exercise itself, your body has to work to keep you stable so you don't end up on the floor. It's also a great leveler – you will soon find out if your right side is stronger than your left, or if, despite your strength, you are sorely lacking in balance and coordination. In general, a 22 inch ball is perfect if you are under 5 ft 4 inches – otherwise, you need a 26 inch ball. The thing to look for is a ball that, when you sit on it, supports your hips slightly higher than your knees. Pump it up nice and firm.

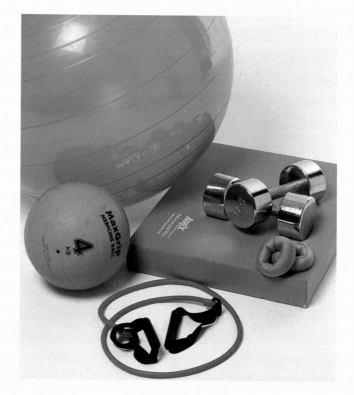

Medicine balls are also making a comeback in modern gyms, probably due to the surge of popularity of one-to-one training. You can't get quite so much out of medicine ball workouts on your own (as many of the best moves involve catching, passing, and throwing) but they can add challenge to abdominal moves and are good for more explosive speed work.

Resistance tubing – with or without handles – has many advantages. It takes up hardly any space, you can easily manipulate the resistance by creating more or less tension in the band, it is inexpensive, and offers a great alternative to dumbbells and machines but there are some limitations. One idiosyncracy of resistance tubing is that the hardest bit of the move is at the end of the range while, if the same move is performed with a dumbbell, the toughest bit is in the middle of the range (often described as the 'sticking point'). It also isn't possible to perform every type of exercise with tubing providing the resistance, simply because you can't get the direction of the movement to work against gravity. A simple, cheap addition – a door attachment, which allows you to hook the tube over a closed door frame – expands your repertoire considerably. Exercises using a range of equipment (and no equipment at all!) are offered in the *Weights for Weight Loss* workouts.

Working order

As the ACSM guidelines stress, strength exercises need to be cleverly sequenced. In other words, don't work your muscles in a random order. Individual exercises are often described as either 'compound' or 'isolated.' A compound exercise is one that uses lots of muscle groups to execute the action (such as a squat) while an isolation exercise hones one specific muscle or muscle group (like a hamstring curl). In order to get the most out of every exercise, it's important to structure your workout so that you start with the multi-muscle exercises and then narrow in on the more isolated moves. For example, you'd do push-ups before you did triceps pushdowns.

Even if you are doing mainly isolated muscle group exercises, think big to start with and work down to the smaller muscles. Another good principle to factor in is to alternate a pushing move with a pulling one. For example, if you've just been pulling in a seated row, follow it with pushing in a chest press. Bearing in mind the importance of rest, you can also alternate upper and lower body exercise to allow the muscles to recover without squandering your time – but remember to still employ the other principles outlined above. A recent study from Brazil found that, whatever order muscles are worked in, the final exercises in a workout tend to be the poorest – so don't let those big, calorie-hungry muscles off the hook by saving them till last!

Many fitness practitioners recommend that the abdominal muscles are trained last, since

BODY TYPES AND WAYS TO WORK OUT

The advice relates to the somatypes described in Chapter 3. It is just a guideline and should be read within the context of the rest of the information in this chapter.

Mostly ectomorph

Use weights that you can lift only six to ten times and rest for at least two minutes between sets. Train at least three times a week, focusing on compound movements to recruit multiple muscle groups with each exercise. Train consistently, too, as any strength you gain will be harder to hold on to than for other body types. It's also wise to change your program regularly.

Mostly mesomorph

Mesomorph guys are the kind who just walk into the gym and gain muscle. As a woman that is less likely to happen but you will probably find that your body responds very quickly and visibly to weight training. If you have the classic broad-shouldered, narrow-hipped mesomorph shape, focus on the lower body to prevent looking too muscular up top. Or, to get the physiological benefits of strength training and aid weight loss without gaining size, you could focus on muscular endurance as opposed to strength. By doing lots of repetitions, you get all the fibers involved through a process called 'motor unit rotation' (basically, the knackered ones move aside to let the fresher ones do the work). Aim for twenty to thirty repetitions, moving swiftly from exercise to exercise and set to set with little rest. Please note, though, that this does not constitute pure strength training.

Mostly endomorph

Endomorphs don't find it as easy as mesomorphs or as hard as ectomorphs to build muscle. Use moderate weights that you can lift nine to fifteen times at a swift training pace (allowing 1 minute rest between sets and exercises). Train two or three times a week, and focus on shaping the upper body to create balance to a pear-shaped lower half.

they are needed to provide stability and support throughout all the other exercises, although some argue that working them beforehand will 'switch' them on so that they function more efficiently during subsequent exercises. You don't have to do all your abdominal and core stability work at once, anyway. You could start with some simple exercises to warm up and switch on the core stabilizers and then complete your abs workout at the end of your strength training regime. The best advice is to experiment and find what works best for you. If you have a lower back problem, however, you should definitely do them at the end so that you have sufficient core strength to support the spine during your workout.

Talking technique

To get the longest leanest look your body will allow, you need to work through the full range of motion of each particular joint in your strength training. Continually working in a shortened range can actually cause the muscles to drop sarcomeres (the little 'blocks' that each muscle fiber is made up of) and become physically shorter and therefore bulkier. Working through a full range enhances strength development too. A study published in 2005 in the *Journal of Strength and Conditioning Research* compared the progress of women training through a partial range and a full range and found that the latter was far superior.

One of the best ways to ensure good technique is to watch yourself perform the exercise in the mirror. I know some people hate to do this but it really can be helpful in allowing you to see and feel correct posture simultaneously and store that information. Another important consideration is to know what muscle groups you are working, where they are and what the movement is that they are meant to be executing. I don't think I have ever been to the gym without spotting someone performing an exercise so badly that it is a complete waste of time.

Regardless of what muscle group you are working, I think it's a good idea to focus on your core muscles. Using your core will make executing the movement easier, it will protect your back from injury and make the core muscles themselves stronger and more efficient.

As for speed of movement, the usual advice is to ensure each repetition takes about two seconds on the lift and four on the lower and the whole exercise is performed with control. But this isn't always the ideal. If, for example, you were aiming to improve your explosiveness in a muscle group (say, to aid your leaping height in netball or your dive in squash) then the SAID principle comes into its own: the notion that you get what you train for. In that scenario, a more rapid motion would be better. There is no harm in experimenting with speed of movement, provided you maintain control and don't use momentum to swing the weights.

Breathing

Breathing is a Very Good Idea when you are strength training! Yet many people automatically hold their breath when they move a weight around. Try not to acquire this habit, even if you can't quite master the commonly recommended breathing rhythm of exhaling on the effort and inhaling on the release. The important thing is to get oxygen into your lungs and get carbon dioxide out. And bear in mind, you may well find lifting weights easier if you can learn to exhale on the toughest bit of the movement.

Some experienced weight lifters and bodybuilders use a technique called the Valsalva Maneuver when lifting exceptionally heavy weights. This technique enables the weightlifter to increase the pressure within the abdominal and chest cavity by forcibly breathing out while keeping the throat closed to trap and pressurize air in the lungs (sorry to be graphic but like when you're trying to have a poop when you are a kid). This maneuver should most definitely be avoided in weight training as it sends blood pressure soaring, can cause dizziness or fainting and is positively dangerous for those with existing high blood pressure or cardiovascular disease.

Putting a routine together

So let's start to put the framework for your weight-training regime in place. There are six main considerations:

- How much am I going to lift?

- How many reps and sets will I perform?

- How much rest will I take?

STRONG WORDS

WHEN IS ONE-SET TRAINING WORTHWHILE?

If you are a total beginner, it seems that one set will suffice to make significant strength gains. A study from Appalachian State University found that almost any overload at all could instigate change in subjects who were totally inexperienced at strength training). In addition, one-set training has been shown to be sufficient to offset the loss in muscle tissue associated with losing weight. Research published in the journal *Medicine & Science in Sports & Exercise* found that adding one-set strength training to aerobic exercise and diet attenuated muscle loss while still allowing fat loss to take place. And finally, if your main goal is to develop your aerobic fitness (say, for example, you are training for a half marathon or a charity bike ride), one set may be enough to create a base of muscular strength and more robust connective tissues. It is worth mentioning that one-set groups in research studies do get stronger just not as strong as the multiple-set groups. For example, in one study they gained 6% in thigh strength compared to 15% for the multiple-set group.

- How often will I train?

- What exercises will I do?

- How will I progress?

Before giving the advice that follows, I think it's worth pointing out that there does have to be a certain amount of experimentation in this. Not everyone will get the same physiological response to a set protocol. If you aren't seeing results, look at changing what you are doing to see if that works better. But only change one thing at a time and stick with it for three to four weeks – change everything at once and you won't know what worked… or didn't.

Load, reps, sets, and rest explained

The issue of how much weight to lift, how many times to lift it, and how much rest to take are all interrelated. Lifting the heaviest load you can manage, for example, will probably mean lifting it just three to four times and taking lots of rest, while a weight that is only half of what you could ultimately shift could be lifted more times and wouldn't necessitate so much rest. Strength specialists use percentages of what's called the 'One Repetition Maximum' (1RM) to define how heavy the load should be to gain a particular result. The 1RM is the heaviest weight you could lift once (theoretically, at least, as it's not always easy to measure). So 80% of 1RM is a weight that equals 80% of the weight you could lift only once.

Throughout this book I shall talk about 'sets' and 'reps' to refer to the number of times you do an exercise. A rep or repetition simply means lifting and lowering a weight once. A set is a pre-determined number of reps which you might do just once or repeat a number of times with a rest between each set.

Doing the numbers

Studies have found that working at 80+% of the maximum load is best for strength and power, while general muscular hypertrophy (growth) involves working at 60–80% of IRM, but with a greater overall volume of reps and sets. Working below 60% of 1RM has been shown not to increase strength at all, although it will build muscular endurance.

But how does that relate to actual numbers of repetitions – and numbers of sets? (This is useful to know as it removes the necessity of having to test out your IRM in every exercise.) Research suggests that six or fewer reps provide the most strength and power gains, while six to twelve reps produce strength and size gain. In a study from Goethe University, subjects did three sets of just six to nine repetitions but at an effort level at which they couldn't actually perform another repetition, and gained significant strength. Beyond 20 repetitions, you are looking at predominantly endurance gains. Remember, though, that muscles can't count. So don't do a specific number just because you said you would. If your technique has gone AWOL before you've finished the planned set, then stop.

Is one set enough?

Not so long ago the virtues of 'single set' training were widely extolled but recently the tide has turned and generally – as concluded by a largescale study at the University of Queensland – multiple sets are a better bet. A study in the *Journal of Strength and Conditioning Research* from Appalachian State University found that, in untrained women, multiple sets yielded greater strength gains and other positive adaptations than single-set training. In the Goethe University study women with basic weight training experience gained more strength after a three-set program compared to a one-set program. What's more all the subjects in the study performed the same number of repetitions and the same exercises, making comparisons between one and three sets clear and simple.

STRONG WORDS

HOW LONG WILL IT TAKE TO SEE RESULTS?

In previously untrained people, eight to twelve weeks is needed to see changes in actual fiber size. Initial improvement in strength is largely attributed to better nerve-muscle communication but it's also due to more efficient help from 'synergist' muscles (those that assist the movement) and increased inhibition of opposing or 'antagonist' muscles – so that they don't impede the working muscle's contraction.

As far as fat loss – and increased muscle gain – is concerned, the volume of training you do plays a part in maximizing calorie expenditure, so the more 'work' you do the better. One of the key factors in improving strength is that the muscle needs to be fatigued in order to trigger the physiological mechanisms that cause size and strength gains. Fatigue is much greater in multiple set protocols. Secondly, research shows that we reach maximum power in the second or third set of an exercise, not the first. Traditionally, multiple sets means three but there's no reason to stop there – four or five sets may be beneficial, depending on your personal goals and needs.

And the rest

In general, the higher the percentage of your 1RM you are working at, the longer the rest period between sets should be. Insufficient rest means optimal effort cannot be put into the next set, while too much rest deactivates the muscle. In the Goethe University study, the rest interval between sets was two minutes. The researchers suggest that the protocol they used may have improved strength because the two-minute rest meant that the second and third sets took place under a certain amount of prefatigue, triggering motor unit rotation, whereby the tired muscle calls in more motor units to help with the workload, as those already used in the first set are whacked.

The inclusion of more motor units increases the overall stress on the muscle and also, due to the activation of a larger number of nerves,

improves neuromuscular efficiency, which has a bearing on strength. If you don't want to waste time hanging around between exercises, you can, of course, use your rest time to work on a completely different muscle group, to allow the worked one to recover.

The general principle to follow is that the higher the number of reps you are doing, the more you are focusing on endurance and, therefore, the shorter the rest period should be – perhaps 45–60 seconds. The fewer reps you are doing the heavier the weight and the more important it is to make a full recovery for the next set. You may therefore be looking at as much as three to four minutes' rest between sets. If you are working in the middle range – say, six to ten reps – to gain both strength and some firmness and growth – I recommend that you allow two minutes' rest between sets.

What's the frequency?

So you've decided on reps and sets – you know what weight you are going to lift. How many times a week are you going to get with the program? As we've seen, the ACSM recommends two to three times per week for beginners and intermediates – and up to five days per week for advanced exercisers. A study from the University of Alabama looked at the relative strength gains of a group of subjects who worked either one day a week, performing three sets to failure, or three days a week, with one set to failure. On upper and lower body strength the three-day a week group achieved greater gains in strength and lean body mass implying that, although the total exercise volume stayed the same, the more frequent training was more successful. But the differences were not that great (the one-day a weekers gained 62% of the strength that the three-day a weekers did) and the researchers also found that the more experienced a subject is in strength training, the more the emphasis needs to be placed on volume.

A baseline frequency of two sessions a week seems to allow existing gains to be maintained. What is perhaps most surprising about the results of this study, though, is the fact that even *one* day a week of training made such a significant difference to strength gains. Even if you can't commit to three or more sessions, the evidence shows that strength training is far from a waste of time.

More isn't necessarily better

Incidentally, if you *do* choose to train more frequently, it is possible to have too much of a good thing. The body needs 48 hours to recover and adapt to the stress of the training you have placed upon it. So do not strength train the same muscle group on consecutive days. If you do, then you take away the 'window of opportunity' that your body has to make the necessary repairs and changes in order to cope with that same workload next time round. There is no need to train any muscle group more than three times a week. You can still train daily, but ensure that you alternate between different muscle groups to allow each one to come to the next training session refreshed.

STRONG WORDS

GETTING PERSONAL

A study in the journal *Medicine & Science in Sports & Exercise* showed the value of a personal trainer in getting the most out of strength training. Over twelve weeks, subjects who were supervised increased their workload more considerably than unsupervised subjects, and made greater gains. It's worth investing even in one or two sessions to ensure you are getting the technique right, if you can't – or don't want to – go the whole hog.

This is what is known as a 'split routine' – where you turn up to train, say, the shoulders, chest, and triceps on Mondays and the legs, back, and biceps on Tuesdays. Whether you adopt a split routine or not is largely determined by how much time you want to spend in the gym. It's fine to train the whole body in one session, each time you work out, if you prefer to do so.

Anything goes!

Before we leave the *how much, how often, how hard?* question behind, what is perhaps most crucial to remember is that almost *anything* works, at least initially. And, interestingly, it is as you become a more experienced strength trainer that variety – in intensity, volume of training, speed of movement, and exercise choice – becomes even more important in continuing to reap benefits.

Exercise choice and making progress

So let's now think about choosing the right exercises to perform. Since the goal is to increase lean muscle mass, calorie expenditure and, hopefully, maximise metabolic rate and afterburn – we want to emphasize those compound or multi-muscle group exercises. After all, the more muscles that need to get involved, the harder we are working and the more energy we are expending. We also, presumably, don't want to spend seven hours a week working out with weights, so using compound exercises is more time-efficient. But there are always specific muscle groups that we want to tone up so, in addition to the twelve main moves in the *Weights for Weight Loss* workouts, there are targeted toning segments that focus on tightening and shaping some of the classic problem areas. These also offer you some variety as you progress – as you can swap exercises from the main workout for targeted toning moves – or add in a few of the latter for a more challenging and longer session.

In order to make continued successful progress, it's a good idea to use the periodization strategy described in the ACSM guidelines (see page 36). In other words, you apply progressive overload logically, rather than randomly.

The first step in a periodized program is to lay the foundations on which you intend to build. That is why I recommend you embark on your strength training journey with the 'Foundation Workout.' Follow it for two to six weeks, depending on your existing fitness level, before moving on to the *Weights for Weight Loss* workouts. You'll find out more about how to progress beyond the twelve-week programs later on.

Warming up

Regardless of the number of reps and sets you plan to do, you should always start your weights workout with a warm-up. It doesn't need to take long – and the benefits you'll reap make it well worth it – your muscles will work more efficiently when they are warmer, be less prone to injury, according to a study published in the *American Journal of Sports Medicine*, and quicker to recover.

The first part of the warm-up aims simply to increase heart rate and body temperature – it's the 'get things moving' phase…. If you are in the gym, a few minutes walking on the treadmill, rowing, stepping, or cycling will do the trick. Otherwise, brisk marching on the spot, with some side steps and knee bends, is fine.

Then, in the second phase, mobilize (circle, bend, extend) your major joints by taking them gently through their full range. Start with the neck, then the shoulders, trunk, hips, knees, and ankles. Finish by gently mobilizing the back.

Don't stretch your muscles before your weights workout. There is evidence that stretching prior to exercise actually reduces force output for up to an hour. But prior to each exercise you perform, it's a good idea to 'rehearse' the exercise with no weight at all or a very light weight, just to gear up the neuromuscular pattern involved.

Cooling down

Strength training differs from aerobic exercise in that heart rate doesn't remain elevated for a prolonged period – it rises and falls because you intersperse work with rest. So a cool down to gradually take the body back to a 'resting state' isn't really necessary. However, it *is* important to stretch. At the very least, this helps restore muscles to their natural resting length following a period of intense activity. And if you do it correctly, and often enough, it will also help you improve your range of motion and increase suppleness.

Stretching know-how

Do you find that despite doing your stretching, your flexibility never seems to get any better? If so, it may be that you aren't following the golden rules, in terms of how far to stretch, how long to hold it and what technique to employ. Recently revised American College of Sports Medicine guidelines suggest 15–30 second holds are needed and that each stretch should be repeated two to four times. (In other words, those slap-dash four-second stretches that we are all occasionally guilty of won't contribute to flexibility!) Flexibility also varies from joint to joint – you may have fantastic range of motion in your neck and shoulders, for example, while your hamstrings are as tight as guitar strings. Or you may be more flexible on your right side than your left. Whatever the case, work harder on the less flexible muscles and stiffer joints otherwise you'll simply maintain your imbalances.

Your muscles should always be warm when they are to be stretched, so if you are not slightly warm, breathless, and sweating, then spend a few moments raising your heart rate and body temperature again with some gentle aerobic exercise. Stretch until you feel tension and a slight 'irritation' in the muscle but not pain. As the muscle relaxes, you can move slightly deeper into the stretch and hold again. Use your breath to help you develop the stretch: inhale as you ease off, and exhale as you move deeper into the stretch. Do not bounce in and out of your 'end' position, however.

Finally, do it after *every* session. Not just once in a blue moon…. The ACSM guidelines recommend stretching a minimum of two to three days a week, with five to seven days being the ideal.

The post-strength training stretch

The following routine addresses all the muscles you'll be working on in the Foundation and *Weights for Weight Loss* workouts. Hold each position for 15–30 seconds (per side, if appropriate) and perform each stretch twice. Add 1–2 repetitions on the tight side if there is a noticeable discrepancy between left and right.

1 HAMSTRINGS

Stand face on to a support between knee and hip height. Extend one leg and place it on the support, with the foot relaxed. Your supporting leg should be perpendicular to the floor. Now hinge forward from the hips (keep the arch in your lower back), with the pelvis level and the knee of the extended leg straight. Feel the stretch along the back of the supported thigh. To emphasize the outer hamstring, bring the leg slightly across the midline of your body and rotate the hip joint slightly inwards. To emphasize the hamstrings closest to the middle of the body, turn out at the hip joint and take the leg slightly away from the midline of the body. Finally, bend the knee slightly to emphasize the belly of the muscle. You don't need to pull your toes back toward you – the only reason this intensifies the stretch is because it stretches the sciatic nerve, too.

2 UPPER AND LOWER CALVES, FEET, AND ANKLES

Stand facing a support, with feet a stride length apart, back leg straight, and front leg bent. Press the back heel into the floor so that you experience a stretch in the middle of the calf muscle. Turn your toes slightly inwards to focus on the outer side of the calf. Hold. Now bring the back leg forward a little, bend the knee, and flex the hips, so that the stretch moves down to the lower part of the calf and Achilles tendon. Finally, with both legs still bent, place the toes of the front foot up against the support to stretch the muscles along the sole of the foot.

QUADS

3 Stand tall with feet parallel. Lift your right foot, taking your right hand behind you to grab it and bring it toward the bottom. Bring the pelvis into a neutral position and gently press the foot into your hand, keeping the knees close together. It doesn't matter if your stretching thigh is in front of the supporting one, as long as you feel a stretch.

4 INNER THIGHS

Sit on the floor with your knees drawn into your chest and feet flat on the floor. Drop the knees out to the sides and use your elbows to gently press the legs open. Don't round the back, sit up tall. If necessary, sit on the edge of a rolled-up towel to prevent your back rounding. Hold, then extend the legs out to the sides and hinge forward from the hips.

5 HIPS/GLUTES

Sit against a wall with your legs outstretched.
Cross your left foot over your right thigh and put
the foot flat on the floor. Now place your right
arm around the left knee and gently pull it
around toward the right shoulder (rather than
hugging directly to chest), sitting up tall.

6 HIP ROTATORS

Lie face up on the floor and bring one knee into
your chest, leaving the other leg flat on the floor.
Now grasp the ankle of the bent leg and holding
the knee in place with your other hand (like a
hinge), gently pull the ankle toward you until you
feel a deep stretch in the hip area of the lifted leg.

7 SIDE STRETCH (OBLIQUES, QUADRATUS LUMBORUM)

Stand with your feet below the hipbones and arms above your head, hands interlinked. Drop the torso directly to the right side (as if you were sandwiched between two plates of glass), keeping the core engaged and the arms stretching upwards. Feel a stretch along the left side. Pause, then return to the start position and sink down to the left side.

8 CHEST (PECTORALIS MAJOR)

Stand with your feet below the hipbones, with your hands interlinked behind you, palms facing each other. Keeping the shoulders back and down, draw the arms away from you, until you feel a stretch along the front of the chest. If you don't feel a stretch through this action, do the chest stretch on page 61...

9 UPPER BACK (LATISSIMUS DORSI, RHOMBOIDS, TRAPEZIUS)

Stand with your feet below the hipbones and knees bent – clasp your hands together in front of the body, palms facing you, and push the arms away from you, feeling a stretch along the back of the shoulders and upper back. Try to make your upper back into a 'C' shape as if you were resisting being pulled forward by your hands and your knees.

10 BACK OF UPPER ARM (TRICEPS)

Raise your right arm overhead and allow it to drop down behind your back. Now take the left hand up to the right elbow and gently push the arm back until you feel a stretch along the back of the right arm. Swap sides.

11 FRONT OF UPPER ARM (BICEPS)

Stand side on to a wall in a split stance with the leg closest to the wall in front of the other. Place your right hand against the wall at shoulder height, with the fingers pointing backward. Now, keeping the hand pressed firmly against the wall, lean forward until you feel a stretch along the front of the arm from shoulder to wrist. Swap sides.

12 SHOULDERS (DELTOIDS)

Bring your left arm across the body, just below shoulder height, and use your right hand (holding above the left elbow) to gently press the arm across the chest. Don't hunch the shoulder up. Swap sides.

13 NECK (STERNOCLEIDOMASTOID, SCALENES, SPLENIUS)

Stand tall and take your head directly to the right side, not allowing it to tilt upward or downward. Then rotate the head to the right and drop it forwards. Change sides.

14 HIP FLEXORS (ILIOPSOAS)

From a lunge position, with the right foot forward, take your left knee to the floor with the lower leg extended behind it (the knee well behind the hip) and the toes facing down. Tighten the tummy muscles and extend forward from the hips, until your right knee is at 90 degrees. You should feel a stretch along the front of the hip joint and thigh.

15 LOWER BACK AND ERECTOR SPINAE MUSCLES

Kneel on the floor with a couple of cushions or a pillow on your lap. Bend the torso forward, walking your hands out in front of you and taking your buttocks back to rest on your heels. Let the cushions support the front of the body so that the spine can really flex and stretch out.

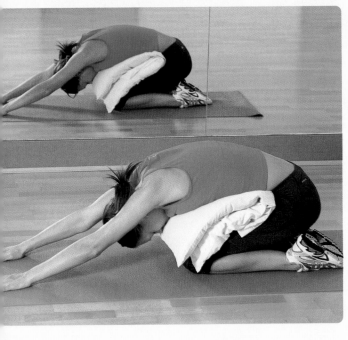

WEIGHTS FOR WEIGHT LOSS WORKOUT

Time to put words into action and start getting stronger, firmer, and slimmer.

This section of the book is where we put the principles of strength training into practice – you'll find a choice of workouts to suit your needs and preferences and to offer variety but they all have one thing in common: results! In order to track your progress, you are going to need some idea of your starting point. Taking a few simple measurements will help you gauge your progress over the next few weeks and months. But *please* bear in mind, not all the benefits you reap from weight training will be immediately noticeable or measurable.

Measurements to take

Make a note of your results, as well as the date you took the measurements...

Weight

It's fine to weigh yourself, but remember that muscle weighs more than fat so even as you lose body fat, you may not end up lighter on the scales.

Body fat percentage

This is optional as you will need to get it measured professionally at a gym, health center or perhaps at your doctor's. Bear in mind that the two most commonly used measurements, skinfold girths and bioelectrical impedance assessment (BIA – where a mild elecrical current is sent through the body) both have wide margins of error. To minimize this, get the same person to take skinfolds each time you get measured and get your BIA reading done when you are well hydrated and at the same stage of your menstrual cycle each month.

Girths

WAIST – Measure around the narrowest part of your midriff at the end of a natural exhalation.

NAVEL – Measure around the midriff directly over the bellybutton.

HIPS – Measure across the top of the buttock cheeks.

THIGHS – Measure 8 inches up from the top of your kneecap and take a circumference measurement of your thigh.

UPPER ARM – Measure 4 inches up from your elbow crease and take a circumference measurement.

Building a firm foundation

The Foundation Workout is the starting point for all newcomers to strength training – and those who haven't exercised for a while. It's all about working from the inside out, serving as a stepping stone to the more challenging workouts that follow. Don't be disheartened that little or no weight is used in the exercises – it is because they are working the 'tonic' muscles of the body, whose role it is to support, stabilize, and protect the joints when the larger, more dynamic (phasic) muscles are

DOING THE FOUNDATION WORKOUT

• Warm up first.

• Wear something loose and comfortable.

• Breathe freely throughout.

• Use an exercise mat ideally or at least a thick towel or rug to support the spine.

• You will need a resistance tube or band, a step or stair, a wall, and a cushion or rolled-up towel.

• Build up gradually to the number of reps and sets suggested if you can't do it straight away.

• Do the exercises in the order shown.

• Rest for 30 seconds between sets EXCEPT for on the stretches, in which there is no need to take a rest. On some moves you can use the rest time to work the other side of the body so that you don't waste time.

called into play. The goal is to improve their responsiveness and muscular endurance rather than their brute strength.

At the very least, this workout will improve your posture, enable you to move more gracefully, help ease muscular tension or joint pain, and help redress imbalances. And best of all, it will ensure you get the best possible results from your strength training program. Before you start, recap on the three steps to better body awareness on page 29.

The foundation workout

The rotator cuff muscles

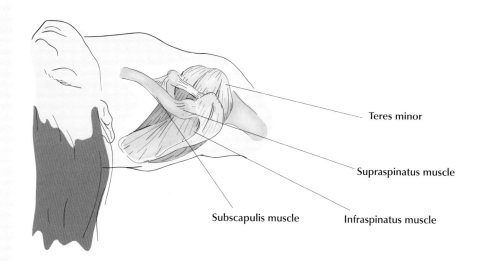

Teres minor

Supraspinatus muscle

Infraspinatus muscle

Subscapulis muscle

1 ARM HINGE

What's the point?
The rotator cuff is a group of small postural muscles that serve to stabilize the shoulder joint, like guy ropes around a tent. Strengthening them will reduce the overpowering of the larger muscles, help protect your shoulder joints when you lift weights, and improve your shoulder position, preventing impingement and contributing to better posture.

How to do it:
1 Take a resistance band and hook it around a closed door handle, or something else sturdy of a similar height. Take a few steps away so that the band has some tension and position your arm so that the upper arm is close to your side and the forearm at a right angle across your body.

2 Now, 'set' your shoulder blades and open the chest. Pulling against the resistance, 'hinge' the arm open to the side, keeping the upper arm close to the torso. Pause then return to the start position and repeat until you complete the set.

3 Now turn around so that the resistance is coming from the other way (i.e. your arm is in the 'open' position at the start…

4 …and the resistance comes when you bring it across the body). Again, ensure that you 'set' your shoulder blades – and align your upper back and shoulders before you start. Use a maximum pain-free range of motion.

How many?
Do 2–4 sets of each position – 8–10 reps per set on each side.

2 HEAD AGAINST A BRICK WALL

What's the point?
To strengthen the 'thoracic extensors,' the muscles that maintain the natural curve of the upper spine, and counteract 'protracted head syndrome,' an unhappy combination of neck flexion, head extension, a concave chest, and rounded shoulders!

How to do it:
1 Stand a few inches from a solid wall and rest your back, shoulders, and head against it.

2 Now push off, so that only the back of your head is in touch with the wall but still in line with your spine. You may feel as if you have created a double chin, but that's OK! Keep your shoulders relaxed and the core engaged.

How many?
Hold for 8 seconds and repeat 5 times.

3 CALF DROP AND RAISE

What's the point?
To improve lower leg muscle balance and strengthen calf muscles during the lowering phase of movement, where they tend to be weak.

How to do it:
1 Stand on the edge of a step or stair with your feet half on and half off – and holding on to something for balance.

2 Rise swiftly and fully up on to the toes…

3 …then lower yourself down moderately slowly, allowing the heels to drop as far below the level of the stair as they can. This part of the exercise is really important, so go to the end of your natural range of movement. Then rise explosively upwards again and repeat the slower descent.

How many?
Do 3 sets of 15 reps.

TIP: Why not do your chest stretches between sets of the calf drop and raise to save waiting around?

4 CHEST STRETCH

What's the point?
To stretch the shoulder protractor muscles (pec minor, serratus anterior), which pull the shoulders forward and down, giving a hunched posture. It's essential to stretch these before strengthening the opposing muscle group.

How to do it:
1 Stand in an open doorway and take one arm to the doorframe, with the upper arm slightly higher than horizontal to the frame. Now gently lean forward to 'open' the front of the shoulder and chest. You should feel a stretch right into the armpit area. Breathe normally and hold for 30 seconds. Swap sides.

How many?
2–4 on each side.

5 HIP AND THIGH STRETCH

What's the point?
The front of the hip is a classically tight area in women, particularly in those who spend a lot of time sitting down and post-pregnancy. Tight hip flexors pull the front of the pelvis down, throwing the back out of alignment and causing the tummy to protrude.

How to do it:
1 Adopt a lunge position, and drop down on to your back knee, with the foot outstretched, your torso upright and your front leg bent at a right angle. Tilt the pelvis under and lean slightly forward from the hips until you feel a deep stretch along the front of the hip and thigh of the back leg. (The back knee should be well behind the back hip.) Once you feel the stretch, hold the position for 30 seconds – if the tension eases off, take the stretch further. Swap sides.

How many?
2–4 on each side.

6 FACE-DOWN BUTT LIFT

What's the point?
To strengthen the gluteus muscles without aid from the hamstrings – to improve pelvic stability. This also actively stretches the hip flexors.

How to do it:
1 Lie on your tummy with your navel drawn up to your spine and your forehead resting on your hands. Bend your right leg so that the lower leg is at a right angle to the floor.

2 Squeeze your buttock cheeks gently and, pressing the hipbones into the floor, raise the thigh a few inches off the floor. Hold for 10 seconds then lower. Swap sides.

How many?
Do 5 lifts on each side, alternating from left to right.

7 SHOULDER BLADE SQUEEZE

What's the point?
To strengthen the lower half of the trapezius muscle and rhomboids, which depress and retract the scapulae and work the back of the shoulders.

How to do it:
1 Lie on your tummy with your forehead resting on the floor and your arms outstretched to the sides, bent at the elbow at a right angle.

2 Draw your arms off the floor by squeezing the shoulder blades back and down – trying to keep the hands and elbows level. Hold for 5 seconds, lower and repeat.

Once this gets easy, try doing the exercise using wrist or light weights.

How many?
2 sets of 10 reps, increase the load or the length of the hold as you get stronger.

8 ARM AND A LEG

What's the point?
It strengthens the muscles of the lower back in a functional way, because the arms and legs are moving while the back stabilizes.

How to do it:
1 Lie on your tummy in a superman position, with your arms extended overhead and legs out straight. Engage the core and then lift the right arm and left leg simultaneously off the floor. Hold for 3–5 seconds, thinking of lengthening the limbs rather than aiming for height (don't hunch the shoulders), then lower and repeat on the other side.

How many?
3 sets of 10 reps.

9 CORE QUARTET

What's the point?

Improving the strength and function of the 'core' is probably the most important thing you can do to ensure that you progress to weight training safely and effectively. A strong, reactive core will protect your spine whether you are picking a weight up off the floor, squatting, or lifting a weight above your head. These exercises work the transversus and rectus abdominis, obliques, and pelvic floor, helping to flatten your tummy, nip in the waist, and provide a base for the more challenging abdominal exercises in the main workout.

PART I NAVEL TO SPINE HOLD

1 Start on all fours, with weight evenly distributed between your hands and knees. Keep your back long and straight (neck in line with spine) and allow your tummy to relax completely.

2 Now, contract the pelvic floor and begin pulling up and back from the pubic bone to the navel. Picture most of the work being done by the sides of the tummy *below* the belly button. When the whole of the lower tummy is contracted, hold for 8–10 breaths. Rest, then repeat 2 more times. Don't worry if you have to 're-contract' halfway through – and think of using minimal force to sustain the contraction – don't grip.

When this feels easy, do the exercise exactly as above but, once you've contracted the tummy, extend one arm out in front of you, without letting the shoulders, back, or hips change position. Hold for 2 breaths, then lower with control and smoothly lift the other arm. That counts as one rep. Do 3 sets of 4 reps.

PART II BENT KNEE DROPS

1 Now lie on your back with your right leg extended straight out on the floor and your left leg bent, with the foot flat on the floor next to the right knee.

2 Engage the core and then slowly let the bent leg lower out to the side without allowing the pelvis to twist or rotate or the back to move.

How many?
Aim for 2 sets of 8–12 reps on each side.

PART III TOE TOUCHDOWNS

1 Still on your back, lift both feet off the floor until your knees are above your hips with the lower legs bent to 90 degrees. Engage the core to stabilize the spine.

2 Now, slowly lower one heel until it is 2 inches off the floor. Pause, then raise the leg back and drop the other heel.

3 When this feels easy, once you have lowered the heel, begin to extend the leg out in front, as far as you can without allowing any flexion or extension of the spine. Draw the leg back in and repeat on the other side. To ensure the core stays engaged, you can slip your fingertips underneath your lower back throughout this exercise and ensure the pressure remains the same against the fingers throughout.

How many?
Aim for 2 sets of 8–12 reps, or stop when you can no longer maintain the neutral lower back position.

PART IV SIDE BRIDGE

1 Lie on your side with knees and hips stacked and your weight resting on the lower elbow. Bend the bottom leg to a right angle at the knee but keep the hips on top of one another.

2 Now lift your body up so that the weight is supported on the lower part of the bottom leg

and the elbow only. Consciously draw the side of the waist closest to the floor up toward the center of the body. Don't let the bottom stick out and keep your abdominals contracted.

How many?
Do 2 sets of 3 reps on each side, holding each rep for 5–10 seconds.

10 THE OYSTER

What's the point?
To strengthen the hip rotators and stabilizers.

How to do it:
1 Lie on your left side with your left arm outstretched, your head resting on it and both legs bent, feet in line with your bottom. Do a small pelvic tilt so that you reduce the arch in your lower back, keeping the abdominals tight.

2 Now keeping the feet glued together, open the right leg. Only go as far as you can without rolling the pelvis – and hold each raise for 2–3 seconds.

How many?
Do 2 sets of 10–12 reps on each side.

11 LEG LOCKOUT

What's the point?
This exercise helps to strengthen a muscle known as the vastus medialis obliquus (VMO), which aids alignment of the kneecap.

How to do it:
1 Sit on the floor with your left leg extended, the right leg bent, and your hands slightly behind you. Place a rolled-up towel under your left knee and with your leg slightly turned out from the hip, press down on the towel firmly, locking out the knee and aiming to feel the muscle that sits just above the knee cap on the inner side of the thigh contracting. Hold for 5–8 seconds.

2 Once you can do this comfortably, press down on the towel as above and then lift the leg off the ground completely, holding it for 2–3 seconds. Swap legs.

How many?
Do 4 sets of 5 on each side.

12 PELVIC BRIDGE

What's the point?
To strengthen the pelvic stabilizers, lower back and inner thighs.

How to do it:
1 Lie on the floor with the knees bent, feet flat, and a rolled-up towel, or foam ball between your knees. Raise the body up by rolling through the spine enough to allow the pelvis to clear the floor, squeezing the towel with your inner thighs. Visualize your knees moving away from your body. Hold for 10 seconds, then release and repeat.

How many?
Aim for 5–8 reps.

To progress:
Do the same as above, but once your pelvis is raised, alternately extend one leg and then the other, without allowing the pelvis to rock from side to side or the towel to drop. Allow 2 seconds to extend the leg and 2 seconds to bring it back. Do 10–12 reps.

STRONG WORDS

CHANGING TIMES

If you've started training but have yet to see results, don't be discouraged. Research from Ohio and Pennsylvania State Universities has found that physiological changes begin to take place in the muscles as quickly as after four workouts – it's just you can't see them yet. Changes included an increase of testosterone and growth hormone, both involved in promoting muscle gain and fat loss. If, on the other hand, you feel as if you have seen 'too much' in the way of results, worry not. The initial 'puffing' that some people experience after beginning weight training is due to increased carbohydrate storage, which makes the body hold on to more water. Once you get into the rhythm of training this side effect will diminish.

The weights for weight loss workout

The *Weights for Weight Loss* Workout is a simple yet challenging routine involving twelve exercises that will:
• make every muscle firmer and stronger;
• maintain the right balance between muscle groups to ensure you look longer and leaner rather than bulky and muscle-bound;
• boost your daily energy expenditure and preserve or increase your metabolic rate;
• make daily physical tasks feel effortless, improve your energy levels and – above all – help you to lose body fat and keep it off.

One workout – three ways to do it

Since not everyone has a gym on their doorstep, or wants to use one, the workout comes in three forms. Firstly, there is a free weights workout – the 'gold standard' method of training. Then there is the gym-based version, for those who enjoy the training environment of the gym and like the support and familiarity of the machines and apparatus. And finally, there is a home-based version, which uses nothing but your own body weight and a few inexpensive pieces of equipment that you can stow easily. Use 'the rules' on page 34 to ensure you do the workout safely and effectively and use the right weight and number of reps and sets – and to make sure that you keep making progress, and don't get stuck on a plateau.

Lifting safely

I know I have drummed in the importance of good technique when strength training but that goes for when you are actually picking up and putting down weights, too. NEVER bend over with straight legs to pick weights up off the floor or from a low rack. Bend your knees, engage the core and use the glutes to help you straighten up rather than your back. If necessary, pick up the weight with both hands and hold it as close to your body as possible. In lying down exercises, make sure you have a firm grip of the weight before you extend it – particularly if lifting it over your face or head. And, if the dumbbells are the type with removable plates on the ends, ensure the fixtures are secure before using them.

DOING THE FREE WEIGHTS WORKOUT

- Warm up first.

- Wear supportive sneakers.

- Try to breathe out on the effort and in on the release – if you can't get the hang of that then breathe freely throughout.

- You will need dumbbells and barbells of varying or adjustable weight, a weights bench, a step, and an exercise ball.

- Decide on your weights, reps and sets, and rest (see pages 41–45). Remember, whatever weight you choose, it should feel tough by the end of each set.

- Do the exercises in the order shown.

YOU KNOW WHAT?

Research in the *European Journal of Applied Physiology* found that muscle in the upper body responds to strength training more quickly than the lower body. So you'll be getting compliments on your sculpted shoulders before you get them about your streamlined thighs!

Free weights

1 DEAD LIFT

What it works:
It emphasizes the glutes, hamstrings, quads, back, and the core stabilizers.

How to do it:
1 Place a barbell on the floor – with feet below the hips and toes underneath the bar. Squat down, keeping the back long and straight, the core engaged and not allowing the knees to roll in.

2 Grasp the bar, hands wider than your knees, in an overhand grip, and straighten up fully. Exhale forcefully as you straighten. Use the back muscles to keep the shoulder blades retracted and the chest open and focus your gaze forward to avoid crunching the back of the neck.

3 Lower back into a squat until the bar is just below the knees, then straighten up and repeat.

To progress:
Increase the weight

[2] SQUAT

What it works:
Glutes, quads, hamstrings, and calves.

How to do it:
1 Stand with your feet below your hipbones and a dumbbell in each hand.

2 Engage the core and inhale as you lower your bottom back and down (as if you were going to sit on a stool). Keep your knees tracking directly over your feet – don't let them roll in or out. When your thighs are parallel to the floor – or as close as is comfortable for you – pause and straighten up, pressing up through the heels as you push back up to a standing position.

To progress:
3 As your strength improves, it will be more comfortable to use a barbell, resting across the fleshy part of your shoulders, rather than dumbbells. Keep your torso as upright as possible without overarching the back.

3 LUNGE

What it works:
Quads, glutes, hamstrings – the adductors and abductors also work hard to stabilize you.

How to do it:
1 Take a dumbbell in each hand and take a big step forward with the right leg, so that the left heel comes off the floor.

2 Ensure you are balanced and then bend both legs, lowering yourself towards the floor without allowing the body to rock forward (make sure your right knee doesn't extend in front of your foot). Pause when the back knee is almost touching the floor and then push back up and repeat. Focus on the front leg during the lunge exercise, as this is the one you are working hardest. Finish the set, then swap sides.

To progress:
Rather than starting in the lunge position, a forward lunge requires you to start with feet together and actually step straight into the lunge, bending both knees and ensuring your front foot remains in line with the toes.

4 STEP UP

What it works:
Quads, glutes, hip flexors, hamstrings, and calves.

How to do it:
1 Stand in front of a step high enough to allow your knee to bend to a 90-degree angle when your foot is on it. Take a dumbbell in each hand and step up with your right foot, ensuring the whole foot goes on to the step.

2 Bring the left foot up onto the step, then down with the right and down with the left. Continue leading with the right foot until the end of the set. Begin the next set starting with the left foot.

To progress:
Increase the weight.

5 SINGLE ARM ROW

What it works:
Lats, rhomboids, trapezius, biceps, and the back of the shoulder.

How to do it:
1 Stand side on to a weights bench with your hand and knee on the support, back parallel to the floor (neck in line), and a weight in your other hand, arm hanging straight down.

2 Bend the arm to bring the weight up to the front of the shoulder – focusing on using the back to lift the weight. Keep the core engaged and don't twist the body around or move anything other than the working arm. Repeat on the other side when you have finished the set.

To progress:
Increase the weight.

6 BENCH PRESS

What it works:
The chest, shoulders, and the back of the arms.

How to do it:
1 Lie on a weights bench with your core engaged and feet on the floor or, if you feel more comfortable, on the end of the bench, knees bent. Take a barbell and hold it level with the nipple line, arms straight, and palms facing upward.

2 Exhale as you extend your arms to press the barbell up, inhale as you lower the bar to the chest. Don't lock the elbow joints out and don't bring the shoulders forward to aid extending the bar – simply bend and straighten the arms.

To progress:
A chest press using dumbbells is more challenging than a barbell, as you'll need to stabilize the arms through the arc of movement. To make it harder still, press each dumbbell alternately – this requires greater core stabilization.

7 PEC FLY

What it works:
The chest and front of the shoulders. It also uses the biceps isometrically, as they are used to keep the arm almost straight.

How to do it:
1 Lie on a bench with a dumbbell in each hand, arms almost straight above the chest, palms facing each other, and wrists in line with the forearms.

YOU KNOW WHAT?
One study found that for optimal training of the chest, the dumbbell and barbell bench press can be used interchangeably for variety but flys activate the pectoralis major less and should only be used as an auxiliary – not a main – lift.

2 Open the arms out to the sides, as far as is comfortable, then bring them back to the start position.

To progress:
Increase the weight.

8 OVERHEAD PRESS

What it works:
The shoulders, triceps, chest, trapezius, and shoulder girdle rotators.

How to do it:
1 Stand with your back straight and core engaged, with a dumbbell in each hand, resting on the shoulders with palms facing each other.

2 Extend the arms over the head, allowing them to rotate so that when the arms are straight, your palms are facing the front. Keep your trunk tight and don't allow the torso to tip back to assist you. You should be able to see your arms in your peripheral vision as they are raised – don't take the arms behind the line of the head. Pause, then lower and repeat.

To progress:
3 & 4 Using a barbell makes the exercise harder, as you aren't able to rotate the arms as the bar lifts. Also, try performing the exercise with dumbbells but sitting down, and see how much 'back' you unwittingly put into the move when you are standing.

9 REVERSE FLY

What it works:
The middle and upper back, and back of the shoulders. A good exercise to counteract that rounded front shoulder look caused by too much chest work or a forward posture.

How to do it:
1 Lie face down on a weights bench with a dumbbell in each hand and your chin just off the end of the bench, to keep the neck in line with the spine.

2 Take your arms out to the sides, with arms almost straight and, squeezing the shoulder blades together, lift the weights until they are level with your shoulders. Lower and repeat.

To progress:
Increase the weight.

10 BICEPS CURL

What it works:
The biceps in the front of the upper arm.

How to do it:
1 Sit with a weight in each hand, your arms relaxed down by your sides, palms facing inwards.

2 Either simultaneously or alternately, bend the elbows and rotate the arms, to bring the weight up to the front of the shoulder with the palm facing the shoulder. Pause, lower, and repeat.

To progress:
Increase the weight.

11 TRICEPS KICKBACK

What it works:
The back of the upper arm and rear shoulder.

How to do it:
1 Stand right-side on to a weights bench with your right hand and knee on the bench, back parallel to the floor and a weight in your left hand. Start with the upper arm parallel to the body, elbow at a right angle.

2 Keeping the upper arm still, straighten the arm, taking the dumbbell past your thigh. At the end of the range, try to extend the shoulder slightly (allow the arm to go beyond the line of the body). Bend the arm back to the start position and repeat. Swap sides.

To progress:
Increase the weight.

12 BALL SIT UP

What it works:
Rectus abdominis (sixpack muscle!), obliques, and core stabilizers.

How to do it:
1 Lie back on an exercise ball with your feet resting against the join between the wall and the floor for support. Adjust yourself so that your bottom is just off the front of the ball, with buttocks unclenched and your hands either beside your head or crossed over your chest.

2 Contracting the abdominals, raise and flex the upper torso as far as you can without moving the ball underneath you. Pause, then lower and repeat.

To progress:
Increase reps and sets.

Gym workout

DOING THE GYM MACHINE WORKOUT

- Warm up first.

- Wear supportive sneakers.

- Try to breathe out on the effort and in on the release – if you can't get the hang of that, then breathe freely throughout.

- Remember to keep your core engaged. Although the machine is supporting you, don't use this as an excuse to let it all hang out!

- Decide on your weights, reps and sets, and rest (see pages 41–45). Remember, whatever weight you choose, it should feel *tough* by the end of each set.

- Do the exercises in the order shown.

- Remember to adjust the seat height, pad height, and lever length of each machine where necessary.

- Gym machines are fairly self-explanatory and different brands vary in their set-up. For these reasons, exercise instructions are not given but there are some useful technique pointers to follow.

1 LEG PRESS MACHINE

What it works:
Quads, glutes, hamstrings, and calves.

Technique pointers:
Make sure your feet are the same distance apart as your hipbones and that your feet are pointing directly forward. As you bend the legs, don't allow the knees to roll in and get as close to 90 degrees as you can.

2 SEATED LEG CURL

What it works:
Hamstrings.

Technique pointers:
Maintain the curve in your lower back and don't slump in the chair, so that you get maximum range in the hamstrings. The face down lying leg curl is an acceptable alternative: if you use this machine, don't allow the bottom to lift up as the legs bend.

YOU KNOW WHAT?
A whole muscle is always active but the mechanical emphasis differs according to the body's position, which changes the 'line of pull' – the relation of where the body is moving compared to the line in which the fibers travel. That's why a chest press on a flat surface is slightly different from one on an incline or decline bench.

3 CLOCKFACE LUNGE

What it works:
Quads, glutes, hamstrings, adductors, and abductors. (This is included instead of the classic thigh exercise – the leg extension, which can cause excessive force on the knee joint.)

How to do it:
1 Imagine you are standing in the middle of a clockface. With a dumbbell in each hand, take a big step forward (to 12 o'clock) with the right leg, so that the left heel comes off the floor and the knee travels towards the floor. The right knee should bend to approximately 90 degrees but make sure your knee doesn't extend in front of your foot. Pause when the back knee is almost touching the floor and then push back up.

2 Now lunge to 2 o'clock with the right leg, following the same technique pointers as above.

3 Push back up and then lunge to 11 o'clock. Swap legs.

4 ABDUCTOR MACHINE

What it works:
Opening the legs against resistance works the outer thighs.

5 ADDUCTOR MACHINE

What it works:
Closing the legs against resistance works the inner thighs.

Technique pointers:
Use the fullest range of motion you can and use smooth movements – do NOT swing or 'pulse' the legs open and closed.

6 CHEST PRESS MACHINE

What it works:
The chest, shoulders, and the back of the arms.

Technique pointers:
Whether you are using a seated or lying chest press, ensure that the handles are level with your nipple line and your elbows and wrists are in line with each other. Don't protract the shoulder blades as you straighten the arms, keep them drawn back.

7 LAT PULLDOWN

What it works:
Lats, rhomboids, and biceps

Technique pointers:
Use a wide, overhand grip to focus most on the lats. Think of squeezing the shoulder blades together as you lower the bar and don't allow the shoulders to ride up as you straighten the arms. You can bring the bar to the back of the neck or the front of the chest – but taking it to the back requires good shoulder flexibility. In general, the front position is preferable.

7 ALTERNATIVE: ASSISTED PULL-UP

Technique pointers:
The design of this machine means that the higher the weight you select, the easier the exercise. This is because the weight counterbalances your own body weight. This is an excellent exercise not just for the lats but also for the chest, shoulders, upper back, and biceps. Remember to squeeze the shoulder blades together as you pull yourself up. The wide overhand grip best mimics the lat pulldown but you can experiment with a narrow 'palms up' grip to emphasize the biceps.

8 SEATED ROW

What it works:
The upper and middle back, the back of the shoulders, and biceps.

Technique pointers:
To focus on the back muscles, use a 'palms facing' grip; to focus on the back of the shoulders, use a 'palms down' grip and bear in mind that you will need to use a lower weight for this smaller muscle group. Don't allow the back to arch or move backward as you bend the arms. Instead, focus on opening the chest and squeezing the shoulder blades together.

9 SHOULDER PRESS MACHINE

What it works:

The shoulders, triceps, and chest.

Technique pointers:

Sit tall and engage your core while you do this exercise. Don't over-arch the back to help you straighten the arms.

10 TRICEPS PUSHDOWN

What it works:
Triceps.

Technique pointers:
You can use a straight bar, angled bar, or rope to perform a pushdown. Start with your elbows close into your sides, forearms perpendicular to the floor, and wrists in line with forearms. Come back to this position between each rep – don't allow the arms to bend further than 90 degrees.

10 ALTERNATIVE: ASSISTED DIP MACHINE

Technique pointers:
As with the assisted pull-up, the higher the weight you select the easier the exercise. Don't 'sink' into the shoulders as you bend the arms – keep them back and down, and only lower until you reach a 90-degree angle at the elbow. Keep the body properly aligned and core engaged.

11 BICEPS CURL

What it works:
The biceps in the front of the upper arm. (This free-weights version of this exercise is more effective than using a biceps curl machine.)

How to do it:
1 Stand with a weight in each hand, your arms relaxed down by your sides, palms facing each other.

2 Either simultaneously or alternately, bend the elbows and rotate the arms, to bring the weight up to the front of the shoulder with the palm facing the shoulder. Pause, lower, and repeat.

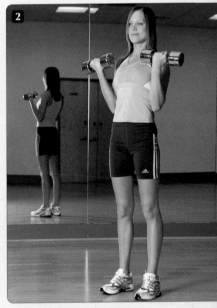

12 AB CURL MACHINE

What it works:
Rectus abdominis and obliques.

Technique pointers:
It's really important to get your position correct in this exercise, so experiment with the seat height and pad position. Don't 'lead' with the head as you curl the torso forward and remember to engage the core. If you don't feel you 'fit' the machine properly, then substitute this move with one of the ab exercises from the Targeted Toning sequence on page 106.

Home workout

DOING THE HOME WORKOUT

- Warm up first and wear supportive sneakers.

- Clear some space before you begin your workout and gather all the equipment you'll need. Have a mirror in the room so that you can monitor your technique and body position.

- You will need an exercise ball, a resistance tube, a chair, an exercise mat, a medicine ball, a balance pad or wobble board, and some dumbbells.

- Do the exercises in the order shown.

- Try to breathe out on the effort and in on the release – if you can't get the hang of that, then breathe freely throughout.

- Some of these exercises use no weight but a change in body position can make the exercise easier or harder.

1 KNEE DRIVE WITH DUMBBELLS

What it works:
Glutes, quads, hamstrings, calves, adductors, and abductors.

How to do it:
1 Stand with your feet under your hipbones with a dumbbell in each hand.

2 Drive up with the right knee, bringing it up to the chest.

3 Then swing it back into a lunge position and immediately drive back up from the lunge into the next repetition. Swap sides.

To progress:
4 Stand in front of a step between shin and knee height (the higher, the tougher) with a dumbbell in each hand.

5 Place your right foot fully on the step and then drive up, bringing the left knee to the chest as you straighten the right leg. Pause, then lower and repeat until the end of the set.

2 SQUAT WITH MEDICINE BALL

What it works:
Glutes, quads, and hamstrings.

How to do it:
1 Stand with your feet below your hipbones and a medicine ball clasped to your chest.

2 Engage the core and inhale as you lower your bottom back and down (as if you were going to sit on a stool). Keep your knees directly over your feet – don't let them roll in or out. When your thighs are parallel to the floor – or as close as is comfortable for you – pause and straighten up, pressing up through the heels as you push back up to a standing position.

To progress:
3 Perform the squat on a balance pad, wobble board, or core board to add an element of instability. Alternatively, use a heavier ball or swap the ball for dumbbells, held at your sides.

3 SINGLE LEG SQUAT

What it works:
Quads, glutes, and hamstrings.

How to do it:

1 Stand tall, next to a support and take the foot furthest from the support off the floor.

2 On one leg, slowly lower your bottom back and down, keeping your weight on the mid-point of the foot, at the back of the arch, and ensuring the knee bends directly over the fourth toe. Allow the torso to tip forward as you bend but keep the back long and straight. This is a tough exercise and no weight is necessary. Swap sides.

To progress:
Increase the reps or slow the movement down.

4 | SIDE STEP-UP

What it works:
The hips, thighs, hamstrings, and glutes.

How to do it
1 Stand side on to a step, quite close to it, with a weight in each hand. Step up with the foot closest to the step…

2 …following with the other foot. Then step down with that foot and follow with the first foot. Make sure the knee is aligned over the toes and keep the body centred as you step up. Repeat on the other side.

To progress:
Increase the weight.

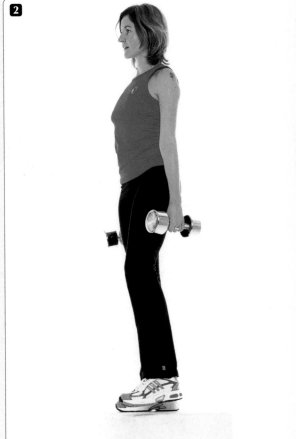

5 HAMSTRING CURL ON BALL

What it works:
Hamstrings, glutes, and lower back.

How to do it:
1 Lie face up with your heels on an exercise ball, legs straight and arms by your sides.

2 Lift yourself up so that your body forms a straight line from head to heels and then, bending your knees, roll the ball in toward your bottom. Pause, then slowly extend it again.

To progress:
3 First, try doing the exercise with your arms crossed over your chest to challenge stability. Then progress to rolling one leg in at a time.

6 PUSH UP

What it works:
The chest, shoulders, triceps, and abdominals.

How to do it:
1 Stand in front of a surface somewhere between waist and knee height (the higher, the easier) and place your hands on the support. Form a straight line from head to toe, with your arms straight and shoulder-width apart or a little wider, abdominals contracted, and head in line with the spine. Lower the body toward the support by bending the arms. When your arms reach a right angle, pause and straighten to repeat.

To progress:
2 Try full push-ups on the floor or place your lower legs on an exercise ball.

7 ANGLED PULL-UP

What it works:

Lats, rhomboids, shoulders, and biceps.

How to do it:

1 Find a sturdy surface that you can get underneath and hold on to (one of those bike parking rails is ideal). Shift underneath the surface and place your feet flat on the floor, legs slightly bent.

2 Grip the surface with an underhand grip and pull yourself up toward it by bending the arms and drawing the shoulder blades back. Pause then lower.

To progress:

Use a lower support.

8 OVERHEAD PRESS

What it works:
The shoulders, triceps, and chest.

How to do it:
1 Sit on an upright bench or chair with your back straight and a weight or an end of resistance tubing in each hand, resting on the shoulders with palms facing each other.

2 Extend the arms over the head, allowing them to rotate so that when the arms are straight, the palms are facing the front. You should be able to see your arms in your peripheral vision as they are raised – don't take the arms behind the line of the head.

To progress:
Increase the resistance or use a heavier weight.

9 BICEPS CURL

What it works:
The biceps in the front of the upper arm.

How to do it:
1 Sit with a weight or an end of resistance tubing (thread the tube under the chair) in each hand, your arms relaxed down by your sides, palms facing each other.

2 Bend the elbows and rotate the arms, to bring the weight up to the front of the shoulder with the palm facing the shoulder. Pause, lower, and repeat.

To progress:
Increase the resistance or use a heavier weight.

10 DIPS

What it works:
Triceps, chest, and shoulder blade retractors.

How to do it:
1 Sit at the front of a sturdy chair with hands on the edge, fingers facing forward. Before you start, depress and retract the shoulder blades.

2 Now shift your bottom off the front of the chair so that your weight is supported by your arms. With your knees bent and feet flat on the floor, lower your bottom by bending the arms. Don't go beyond 90 degrees, and stop when your shoulders start to hunch up or roll forward. Pause and straighten.

To progress:
You can do this exercise with a medicine ball or weight over your thighs.

11 BACK EXTENSION ON BALL

What it works:
The lower and middle back, and glutes.

How to do it:

1 Lie face down on an exercise ball with your feet anchored against the join of the wall and the floor. Adjust your position until your torso is lower than your hips, and put your hands beside your head.

2 Now, using the back and butt muscles, raise the torso up until it is just beyond forming a straight line with the legs. Hold, then lower, and repeat.

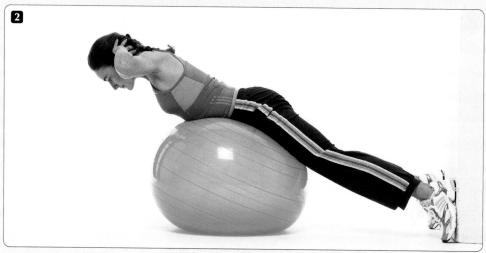

12 BALL ROLL-IN

What it works:
The core stabilizers, abdominals, chest, front of shoulders, upper arms, and hip flexors.

How to do it:
1 Lie face down over an exercise ball, and shunt forwards until just your shins are on the ball, and your weight is supported on your hands, arms shoulder width apart. Contract the abdominals and tilt the pelvis so your back is in a straight line with your legs.

2 Now curl the ball in towards your chest by contracting the abs and rolling the ball towards your torso with your lower legs. Hips should never be below shoulder height – keep your

shoulders drawn back. The movement should be slow and controlled, taking 4–5 seconds each way.

Targeted toning

Any of the exercises below can be substituted for those in the preceding workouts for variety, or in case you don't have the relevant equipment. Alternatively, if you want to home in on a particular muscle group, you can add some or all the targeted toning exercises for that area to your workout.

ABS

1 BALL SIDE RAISE

1 Anchor your feet against the join between the wall and the floor and lie sideways over an exercise ball. The top foot should be in front of the bottom foot and the legs a little bent. Ensure your body is in a straight line.

2 Place your hands beside your ears and, using the muscles at the side of the waist, raise the torso up. It doesn't need to go very far.

[2] BALL REVERSE CURL

1 Lie on a mat with an exercise ball between your calves and the back of your thighs.

2 Engage the core and, gripping the ball with your legs, roll the ball off the floor and toward your chest. Do not use momentum to raise the ball – keep the movements slow and controlled.

3 LEG LOWERING

1 Lie on your back with both legs extended straight up in the air and engage the core.

2 Slowly lower the legs away from the torso, only as far as you can without arching the back. As soon as that happens, draw the legs back to the start, focusing on using the lower tummy to do so, and repeat. You can do this with your legs 12–20 inches from a wall, to prevent yourself going too far. If you like you can also put your fingertips (palms down) under your lower back and use the point at which the back begins to peel away from the fingertips as your cue to raise the legs back up.

4 BALL KNEELING BALANCE

1 Stand in front of an exercise ball. If you are new to this exercise, either get a friend to stand on the opposite side of the ball to help you balance, or have a wall the other side of the ball which you can hold on to if necessary.

2 In a swift movement, put your hands on the ball and rock your body forward to place both knees simultaneously on the ball. Then roll the pelvis forward so that you are in a kneeling up position and take your hands away. You need to constantly adjust your body position to stay balanced – really focus on using the abs, pelvic floor muscles, and glutes to help you.

To progress:
Once you can hold the pose for 30 seconds or so try making tiny figures of eight with the ball, using your core muscles to initiate the movement. When that's easy, try balancing with your eyes shut!

INNER THIGHS

1 SUMO SQUAT

1 Stand with your feet together.

2 Take a large step to the side with knees and hips opening out over the toes. Step back to the start position and repeat on the other side.

To progress:
3 Add a weighted bar across the shoulders or hold a dumbbell in each hand.

2 LEG CROSSOVER

1 Hook one end of a resistance band around something sturdy and loop the other end around your left leg. Shuffle away from the attachment point until there is enough tension in the band, and your left leg is lifted out to the side.

2 Now bring your left leg in towards the center, taking it just across the front of the right leg, toes facing directly forward. Do not allow the hip of the supporting leg to 'dip' and keep the core engaged. Release the leg back to the start position and repeat.

3 CUSHION SQUEEZE

1 This is one you can do anywhere, anytime!
Simply place a cushion, rolled-up towel, or foam
ball between your thighs.

2 Keeping the feet flat on the floor, squeeze
your knees together for a count of 5. Then slowly
release the tension over a count of 5 and repeat.

4 BALL LIFT

1 Lie on a mat with your legs bent and astride an exercise ball.

2 Squeezing the ball between the knees and feet, extend the legs, lifting the ball up, and then lower. This is also a great core stability exercise.

UPPER ARMS

1 NARROW PUSH UP

1 Start on all fours on a mat with your knees behind your hips and your hands below the shoulders, about 6 inches apart, elbows close into your sides.

2 Keeping your neck in line with your spine, bend the arms to lower the chest toward the floor, ensuring the elbows don't 'splay out' but remain close to your sides. Pause, straighten the arms, and repeat.

2 MEDICINE BALL OVERHEAD PRESS

1 Hold the medicine ball in both hands above your head. Stand tall and engage the core.

2 Now keeping the upper arms vertical, lower the ball behind your head by bending the elbows. Only go as far as 90 degrees and then straighten the arms and repeat.

3 RESISTANCE TUBE PUSHDOWN

1 Hook a resistance tube over a sturdy hook or use a door attachment and take an end in each hand, with the elbows close to your sides and arms bent to a right angle.

2 Keeping the shoulder blades pulling together and the chest lifted, straighten the arms, allowing them to go slightly beyond the midline of the body. Pause, then return to the 90-degree position and repeat.

4 TRICEPS KICKBACK

1 Stand side on to a bench, with your left knee and hand supported on it, your back parallel to the floor and one end of a resistance band (or a weight) in your right hand – the other end of the band can be secured with the resting hand. Start with the upper arm parallel to the body, elbow at a right angle.

2 Keeping the upper arm still, straighten the arm, taking the forearm past your thigh. At the end of the range, try to extend the shoulder slightly (allow the arm to go beyond the line of the body). Bend the arm back to the start position and repeat. Swap sides.

HIPS AND BUM

1 SIDE LYING LEG RAISE ON FLOOR

1 Lie on your side with your legs 'stacked' from ankle to hip (directly on top of one another) and your weight supported on your elbow – don't let the body sink into the supporting arm.

2 Raise the top leg a few inches from the supporting one, keeping the toes facing directly forwards. Lengthen the leg out of the hip socket as you extend it. Lower, repeat, and swap sides.

To progress:
Tie a resistance tube around both ankles to create extra resistance (other than gravity) as you lift the leg, or use an ankle weight.

☐2 BALL LEG RAISES

1 Lie face up on your mat, with your feet resting on the ball and hands beside you on the floor. Lift the body off the mat, so that you are in a straight line from shoulders to feet.

2 Get your balance and then lift one foot off the ball, without allowing the pelvis to tilt to the other side. Pause, then lower and repeat with the other leg.

3 SIDE KNEEL

1 Kneel up on a mat and extend your left leg out to the side, keeping your big toe in line with your hip. Using your core muscles, lower your torso to the right and place your right hand on the floor beside you.

2 Now lift the left foot off the floor, keeping it in line with your body.

3 From this position, bend and straighten the knee. Swap sides.

4 BALL DRIFT

1 Sit on an exercise ball and roll down and forward until just your shoulders and head are on the ball. Place your feet hip distance apart. Adjust your position so that your body is in a straight line, using the glutes and abs to stabilize you.

2 Shift your weight over to the right foot, pause, then shift over to the left foot. Continue to alternate for the set.

Making progress

The first six weeks

Focus on technique to establish neuromuscular patterns. Aim for the higher end of your chosen reps, the lower end of your sets ranges and use a slightly lower weight than you optimally can. You can work out the whole body at once or follow a split routine – training each body part two to three times per week.

The next six weeks

To consolidate and build on your gains, move to the lower end of your chosen reps, the higher end of your chosen sets range, and up your weights. Continue to train the same number of times per week. Also feel free to play with different speeds of movement and training techniques (see page 141).

And after twelve weeks?

For maintenance, keep the overall intensity of your training the same (in other words, if you up the weight, decrease the reps) and take the frequency down to twice a week. If you want to continue developing strength, keep frequency as it is, or even increase it. This is the perfect time to add in some new exercises, from the targeted toning workouts, play with different training techniques, and perhaps adopt a split routine. Variety is very important but make sure that it has some kind of logic to it. So if you decide to home in on your upper arms, do it with consistency and progressively build on your gains before moving on to something else.

FUELING YOUR WORKOUTS,

How to get a balanced, healthy diet while you cut calories – and how to fuel up before, during, and after your workouts.

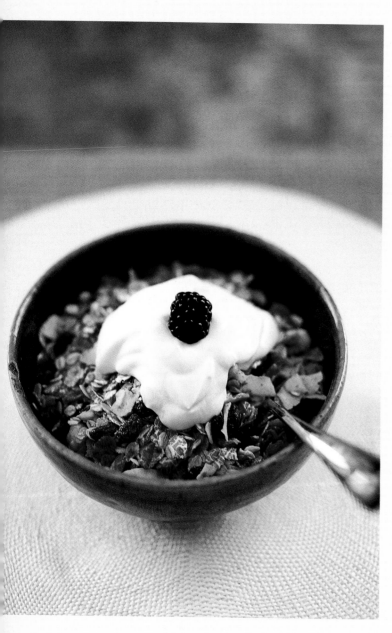

It's common knowledge these days that exercise and diet go hand in hand when it comes to losing weight. But, much as we know this, it can be tough to increase your activity levels *and* reduce your energy intake simultaneously. Often, the problem is simply that we try to reduce calorie intake too much – and to a level that cannot be sustained long term. So guess what? As soon as calorie intake goes back to 'normal,' the weight creeps back on.

The advice contained in this chapter isn't a diet as such, the aim is simply to lay down the ground rules of healthy eating – showing you how to cut calorie intake sufficiently to shed body fat but not so much that you feel deprived or can't keep it up. I am a firm believer that food is one of the great joys in life – far from being just a necessary 'evil' to produce energy in the body. That's why 'soup' diets, meal replacements, and other extreme regimes just don't cut it for me. Do you really want to eat like that for the rest of your life? If the answer is 'no' then you might as well stop right now because the results will last only as long as the diet does.

Losing fat, saving muscle

Research shows that when women diet 25–30% of the weight they shed isn't fat but water, muscle, and even bone. Depressing, huh? And the quicker you lose the weight the

MAXIMIZING WEIGHT LOSS

7

less of it is fat. But strength training changes all that. In a study at Tufts University dieting women were split into two groups – one group just dieted while the other group was put on a strength-training program (twice a week) while they dieted. Both groups lost an average of 13lb during the study but women in the diet-only group lost an average of $^4/_5$lb of lean body mass (muscle) while the women who strength trained actually gained $^2/_5$lb of lean tissue – meaning that every ounce they lost was fat. So you see, once again – weights work for weight loss!

First, let's look at the principles of healthy eating in general. Then we'll explore the ways in which you might consider subtly altering your diet to ensure you get the best results from strength training.

Where should my calories come from?

With the amount of controversy in recent years regarding how much carbohydrate, fat, and protein we should be eating, you could be forgiven for feeling bewildered. While some experts are sticking to their guns and advocating a high-carbohydrate, low-fat diet, others believe that there does seem to be some evidence for reducing carbohydrate intake a little and increasing protein percentage. Still others believe that the burgeoning obesity problem isn't due to too much fat per se, but the wrong *type* of fat. The US Institute of Medicine revised its dietary guidelines in 2002 to recommend a breakdown of between 45 and 65% carbohydrate, 10 and 35% protein,

and 20 and 35% fat (giving much wider margins for all nutrient groups, a lower minimum guideline for carbs and a *higher* maximum guideline for fats). They cite evidence that a high carb, low fat diet can reduce good HDL cholesterol, increase triglycerides, and increase the glycemic load. All undesirable effects. Then again, a high fat diet is linked to heart and cardiovascular disease, obesity, and diabetes. So it would seem that it's a case of what *type* of carbs, fats, and protein you should opt for.

Top class carbs

Most of your daily energy should come from carbohydrate. It is the body's equivalent of four-star fuel. Since only a limited amount can be stored – and since carbohydrate is the only fuel that the brain can utilize without having to convert, supplies need to be constantly replenished. Besides, carbohydrate needs to be present in order for fat to be burned. Carbs also pack a micronutrient-fueled punch – being rich in B vitamins, iron, magnesium, and chromium, as well as fiber, and phytochemicals that can help prevent cancer and promote good health. Experts recommend 4–6g (2.2lb) per kg of body weight per day for people weight training three to five times per week. For a 132lb woman that equals 240–360g per day of carbohydrate.

But carbs vary in their health-giving value. Carbohydrates used to be divided into 'simple' or 'complex' varieties. Simple referred to sugary carbohydrates like table sugar, honey, and fruit sugars while complex meant starchy foods like bread, potatoes, rice, and pasta. The premise was that starches were 'good,' sugars 'bad.' However, surprisingly, there is no

evidence that high sugar intake is related to excess weight – it's only excess calories that can be linked scientifically to excess body fat.

But there is some evidence that the effect of some carbohydrates on the body's insulin levels is related to fat storage. Foods that are high on what is known as the glycemic index (GI) cause a sharp rise in blood sugar, triggering the body to release insulin to get the sugar out of the bloodstream and restore levels to normal. The trouble is, insulin encourages the conversion and storage of the excess sugar as fat. What's more, this sudden surge and then plummeting of blood sugar can cause energy crashes. Low glycemic index foods, in contrast, cause a more gentle insulin response, allowing blood sugar levels to remain more stable – a far preferable state of affairs.

The other point that is often overlooked is that we rarely eat foods on their own and that there are many factors that mitigate the carbohydrate's effect on blood sugar; such as the presence of fiber, fat, protein, acids such as vinegar and lemon juice and the way the food is cooked.

GI IQ

Unfortunately, whether a food is classified as a simple or complex carb doesn't tell you anything about its GI value. So it's a matter of looking foods up. But it isn't possible – or desirable – to base all your nutritional decisions on the GI chart. Otherwise you would be foregoing healthful foods like carrots, potatoes, watermelon, and dried fruit, purely on the strength of their high GI.

In addition, research from the University of Sydney suggests that highly active, fit people have a less pronounced response to high glycemic index foods and so don't have to worry so much about their effects on blood sugar. However, opting for mainly wholegrains, whole-wheat bread, pasta and rice, pulses and beans and eating a wide range of fruits and vegetables should ensure a sustained energy supply as well as a nutritionally rich diet.

Fat facts

There has been a recent shift in expert opinion about dietary fat. While the message for years has been 'eat less fat!' it now appears to be 'eat healthier fats.' Although a gram of olive oil contains the same number of calories as a gram of butter or lard, evidence is increasingly showing that there are some important health benefits to be had from particular types of fat. At present, too much of the fat we eat comes from unhealthy saturated and trans fat sources (derived from meat and dairy products, pastry, fried food, refined and prepackaged products, cakes, and biscuits) and not enough comes from healthier monounsaturated fat (such as olive oil) and sources of the two essential fatty acids, Omega-3 and Omega-6. Aiming to get 12% of your total daily calories from monounsaturated fats, no more than 10% of total calories from saturated fat and a bare minimum of trans fats – will help you maintain a healthy body weight and improve your heart health significantly.

STRONG WORDS

QUALITY NOT QUANTITY

The American Journal of Epidemiology reports that overall carbohydrate intake is not associated with higher body weight, but that processed carb intake is. So steer away from those refined and packaged foodstuffs.

FIVE TOP LOW GI FOODS

• Sweet potato – far lower on the GI than normal potatoes and packed with betacarotene, vitamin C and E – and fiber too.

• Chickpeas – versatile and rich in a phytochemical called saponin which is thought to lower cholesterol.

• Oats – the breakfast of Olympians – oats are high in fiber and energy and can help reduce cholesterol due to the type of soluble fiber they contain.

• Lentils – brown and green varieties are rich in potassium, iron, selenium, and manganese – one study found a preworkout lentil-based meal allowed study participants to keep going for longer than a high GI meal of the same calorific value.

• Grapes – a portable fruit fix that won't send blood sugar soaring. Opt for red ones which are rich in resveratrol, an antioxidant. Fiber-rich skins too.

FAT TYPES

A high intake of saturated fat is linked to heart disease. What's more, saturated fat appears to have no useful role to play in the body so the calories it provides are simply stored as body fat. Major sources include: meat, butter, dairy products, pastry, coconut, and palm oil.

Polyunsaturated fats do have an important role in the body. The two most important types are Omega-6 (linoleic acid) and Omega-3 (linolenic acid). Omega 6 fatty acids may prevent blood clots, help to stabilize blood sugar, and lower blood pressure. But most of us tend to have enough in our diets already. The main source of Omega 6 is any kind of vegetable oil.

Omega-3 fatty acids are the ones we don't tend to get enough of. Consuming Omega-3s is thought to be protective against atherosclerosis (the build-up of fat deposits on the artery walls causing them to narrow), helps to make the blood less sticky, and can lower blood pressure. The major source is oily fish but you can also get significant amounts from some nuts, including walnuts, linseed and its oils, and dark green leafy vegetables, such as kale and spinach.

Monounsaturated fats are found in the oils of the 'Mediterranean' diet. The best-known source is olive oil but rapeseed oil, nut oils, avocados, nuts, and seeds are also good sources.

Trans fats

The effects of trans fats on health are so negative that no 'recommended limit' has been set. In other words, no amount at all is good for you. As well as lowering good HDL, they also raise unhealthy LDL and they have been purported to be linked with certain cancers. That said it can be challenging to avoid trans fats as they are added to so many foods and, in the UK, it isn't a legal requirement to list trans fat content on food labels. Anything in which vegetable oil has been hydrogenated, such as margarine, shortening, fried foods, breads, crackers, snack foods, spreads, processed foods, and ready-meals, contains trans fats.

Reducing fat intake

Most of us eat a higher than necessary amount of fat in our diet regardless of its source (the average British diet contains 41% fat). In addition, many of us consume too many calories overall and so the surplus energy, regardless of where it came from, is converted to fat and stored. Fat, gram for gram, is significantly more fattening than either carbohydrate or protein (containing 9 calories per gram compared to 4 calories for carbs and protein) and just 2–3 calories out of every 100 are used in metabolizing it. Whereas carbohydrate and protein need 6–8 and 25–30 respectively, out of every 100 consumed, to be processed and metabolized.

To lose weight, aim to cut down on fat overall so that around 25% of your total calories come from fat. And ensure that most of the fat you consume comes from the healthier sources (though I am not suggesting you should pile in the olive oil and avocado if you are aiming to lose body fat).

The power of protein

Protein is an essential part of a balanced diet. It helps build and repair all the body's cells, plays a part in the hormonal and immune systems, regulates fluid balance, and is a component of every red blood cell. It also gives structure to our hair, skin, and nails. But, most importantly, it forms the fabric of our muscles. Without sufficient protein you may as well forget about gaining strength or definition in your muscles.

Proteins are constructed from substances called amino acids, of which there are twenty, all with distinctive functions within the body. Of these twenty, eight are termed 'essential' because they must be supplied by the diet and cannot be made from other amino acids.

But what role does protein have in weight loss? Firstly, studies suggest that protein tends to be more satiating than carbohydrate as it spends longer in the stomach. So not skimping on protein means you are less likely to overeat. Secondly, around a quarter of the calories from protein are actually used up in its metabolism. Thirdly, due to its crucial role in repair and maintenance, it is less readily converted and stored as fat. And finally, as we know, one of the consequences of weight loss can be a loss in muscle mass and a subsequent decrease in metabolism and daily energy expenditure. Studies have shown that increasing protein intake to 1.6g (2.2lb) per kg of body weight per day offsets lean tissue loss during dieting. So if you weigh 132lb, that would mean 96g of protein. This may take your protein intake slightly above the normal recommended guidelines but the reduction in

STRONG WORDS

A FAT LOT OF GOOD

Fat is an essential nutrient with an important role to play in a balanced diet. Certain vitamins, including A, D, E, and K are fat-soluble, so can only be derived from fat sources and fat also helps the body absorb those all-important phytochemicals. Secondly, fat produces some important hormones, provides insulation and protection for our bodies and, for women, enables pregnancy and lactation to take place.

fat and carbohydrate intake will ensure that your overall calorie intake does not increase. This extra protein intake is also useful if you are training regularly as the increased breakdown of protein during training needs to be compensated for. This is the case particularly when you are new to exercise as the body has yet to become accustomed to conserving and recycling protein efficiently.

How many calories should I cut for weight loss?

Although many diets recommend cutting 500 calories per day – to create a 3500 calorie deficit in a week (equal to 1lb of body fat) – that could equate to as much as a third or quarter of your total daily energy expenditure. Not only will this feel like a very significant drop in food intake it may also leave you devoid of energy so that your precious training gets pushed aside. A better solution is to cut your daily energy intake by 15%. This avoids the metabolic reactions that take place in response to greater calorie reductions – such as a lower metabolic rate, increased protein oxidation, and depletion of stored carbohydrate in the muscles. Research shows that less than 1200 calories a day triggers hormonal reactions that enable the body to conserve, rather than burn, calories. Therefore the more modest 15% calorie reduction will help you shed fat (rather than water, lean body tissue, and bone) and maintain the loss – without it feeling like starvation!

This begs the question, then, of how many calories you need on a daily basis. There are

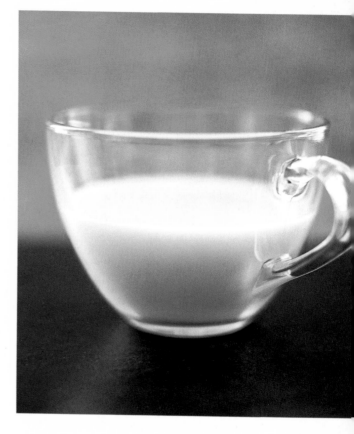

lots of ways of calculating this, based on your resting metabolic rate, weight, age, and so on. The chart opposite will show you how to estimate your own daily energy needs. Once you have the figure, multiply it by 85% to get an idea of how much energy you will be aiming to take in when you cut your calories by 15%.

How much do you need?

How much energy you need is determined by your resting metabolic rate (RMR) plus the amount of extra energy you need to cater for your daily activity.

To get a rough idea of how many calories you need, fill in the following calculations:

1. My weight in kilograms (1 kilogram = 2.2 lb)

2. WOMEN
I am 18–30 years old: weight x 14.7.
Answer + 496 = RMR
OR
I am 31–60 years old: weight x 8.7.
Answer + 829 = RMR

MEN
I am 18–30 years old: weight x 15.3.
Answer + 679 = RMR
OR
I am 31–60 years old: weight x 11.6.
Answer + 879 = RMR

MY ESTIMATED RMR IS ....

3. Take this figure and multiply it by the number below most closely representing your typical daily activity level.

I am totally sedentary	1.2–1.3
I am mostly sedentary (no structured activity, office work)	1.5–1.6
I am moderately active (some walking each day, stair climbing and regular active leisure time activities)	1.6–1.7
I am very active (vigorously physically active each day)	1.8–2.1

MY RESULT IS ....

Making sense of the figures

Remember that you will be burning additional calories through strength training and any other activity that you do regularly. To factor this in, add up the calories expended on exercise during a typical week, divide by 7 and add this to your total. You can get a rough idea of the calorie expenditure of different activities using many website tools, such as www.caloriesperhour.com.

However, it isn't necessary to take in exactly the right number of calories every day. As long as, in general, your intake over the course of a week or so breaks down to your estimated daily requirement you will be fine.

STRONG WORDS

ALCOHOL – THE NON-NUTRITIOUS NUTRIENT

We've talked about the gram for gram content of fat, carbohydrate, and protein – but there's a fourth source of calories in our diets that can add a substantial amount – alcohol. At seven calories per gram it isn't far behind fat in the calorie stakes and a single 'unit' of alcohol contains roughly 8g. The recommended daily allowance for women in the UK is up to three units per day (21 per week) and four units per day (28 units per week) for men. In its entirety this adds between 1100 and 1500 calories to your weekly energy intake. Anyone for a soda water?

More ways to weight loss

- Fidget! Research from the University of Minnesota found that people who couldn't sit still burned 100–500 calories more per day than more sedentary people!

- Eat mindfully. Eating on the move prevents you from noticing that you are eating. Try to sit down and pay attention to the taste, smell, and texture of your food.

- Eat slowly. The hormone peptide YY, located in the intestines, is released when you are full – but it takes a while to kick in.

- Frontload your day. Pigging out at dinner after virtually starving all day results in a lower metabolism. The body is also more responsive to insulin in the morning so is better able to handle carbohydrate without causing a large glycemic response.

- Reduce portions. Even healthy foods are fattening when eaten to excess.

- Boost fiber intake. Fibrous foods keep people feeling full longer and aid weight loss. Fiber also plays a healthy role in digestion by speeding the movement of waste through the intestines, inhibiting cholesterol absorption, and attenuating the blood sugar response.

- Don't set yourself up for failure. Don't try to change everything about your diet at once. Focus on adding in some good stuff before you start subtracting the not-so-good stuff and you won't feel deprived.

Nutrition to maximize the benefits of weight training

There is no doubt at all that the quality and quantity of fuel that you put into your engine affects the performance you'll get. The American College of Sports Medicine's 2000 statement on nutrition and athletic performance confirms that nutrition can affect both performance and recovery in exercise.

What you might need more of...

Protein

The ACSM's statement asserts that protein requirements for active people are higher than average. They suggest that for strength training needs may be 1.6–1.7g per kg (2.2lb) of body weight compared to 0.8g per kg (2.2lb) in sedentary people. But even this amount doesn't necessitate downing loads of egg whites or protein shakes as it is quite possible to get enough protein from your normal diet. For example, if you were looking to take on board 1.4g per kg (2.2lb) per day and you weighed 130lb that would mean 96g of protein, the equivalent of 3/4 cup of milk, a boiled egg, a chicken breast, a cup of baked beans, a small can of tuna, and a handful of peanuts.

Iron

Iron is an essential mineral in the human body – it is involved in the formation of red blood cells and the carrying of oxygen to all the body's cells. Since iron is lost in sweat, and exercise increases sweat, it is more important than ever to get sufficient dietary iron when you are active. Studies suggest that regularly active women need an additional 0.3mg per day on top of the recommended daily amount of 14.8mg per day. Insufficient iron can allow hemoglobin to fall below optimal levels. This is not in itself classed as anemia (which is an iron, rather than a hemoglobin deficiency) but it will hamper your training performance. It is estimated that up to 15% of women are iron deficient – if you think you may be one of them, ask your doctor for a hemoglobin and serum ferritin test. A value less than 12g.dl-1 on the latter is cause for concern.

Carbs

Despite the obvious role protein plays in building muscle carbohydrate is still the fuel of choice for muscles. Exercise physiologists have compared recovery time after exercising to exhaustion with a high protein or high carbohydrate diet. The high protein eaters took five days to replenish their glycogen stores following the intense workouts while the high carb dieters took just two days. What's more, other research found that multiple-set resistance exercise regime resulted in a 25–40% depletion of carbohydrate stores – the higher the volume of training the greater the level of depletion.

Water and fluids

Water, though calorie free and nutritionally empty, is a vital part of our diet. It is involved in every bodily process, from energy metabolism to digestion and muscle contraction, and makes up almost two-thirds of our body composition.

Drinking water (and other fluids) regularly throughout the day is a healthy habit worth having. When you are exercising regularly you need to drink in order to replace fluid lost through sweating. Aim to drink 1–2 cups of fluid 30 minutes before your workout, $1/2$–1 cup every 15–20 minutes during it and 1–2 cups afterwards depending on the length and intensity of the session.

Supplements

The advice on supplements always states that providing you have a healthy balanced diet you don't need them. The exceptions are in the case of:

• Diets low in energy for weight loss.

• Diets in which foods or food groups are omitted due to likes or dislikes.

VEGGIES AND VEGANS

Protein, as we've learned, is the building block for muscle. So a true vegetarian diet presents more of a challenge in ensuring you get sufficient levels. While beans, lentils, nuts, and seeds are high in protein, they are not what are known as 'complete' proteins because they lack some of the nine essential amino acids. Combine them with another wholegrain or vegetable, however, and you can get the full complement of amino acids. The soya bean is an exception in that it constitutes a complete protein all on its own – so eating the bean or its derivatives, like tofu or soy milk, is a smart veggie move.

As far as iron is concerned, providing you eat enough iron-fortified foods, you should get by. Cereals and bread tend to be fortified with iron but always have with orange juice rather than coffee as Vitamin C enhances iron absorption, while caffeine slows it. Also, don't rely entirely on that bag of spinach for, despite being quite abundant in iron, vegetable sources are absorbed at a lower rate than meat-derived sources.

Vitamin B12, part of the B complex, cannot be derived from a vegan diet as it is only present in meat, shellfish, and dairy products. We don't need much – a glass of milk would give you sufficient B12 for the day – but if you don't eat any of the above food groups then you really must take a supplement, containing at least 2mcgs of B12, every day.

- Diets lacking in a particular type of food due to allergy or intolerance.

- Erratic and unbalanced diets.

In these cases a good multi vitamin-mineral supplement is recommended. But what about specific supplements for muscle-boosting, fat-loss enhancing, or joint protection? Do you need them? Do they work? And above all, are they safe? Here are a few for which the evidence is promising…

Conjugated linoleic acid (CLA)

CLA is an essential fatty acid that has been lauded for increasing muscle gain, enhancing fat loss, improving immunity, and even warding off cancer. The evidence in rodents has been utterly compelling but studies on humans have produced more mixed results. Those that have shown a beneficial effect have noted significant changes in body composition (a shift from fat to muscle) when subjects were exercising regularly. In other words, you can't sit on the couch and reap the benefits. No negative effects of CLA supplementation have yet been found.

Recommended dose: 2000–3000mg per day.

Creatine phosphate

Creatine is a protein that occurs naturally in the body and has a key role in the formation of ATP, the body's energy source, particularly to supply short bouts of high intensity activity such as lifting weights. The theory is that boosting creatine levels through taking a supplement enables you to work harder and recover faster, allowing you to do more total work in a session. In studies creatine supplementation has been shown to increase lean body weight but also to increase total body weight (mainly as a result of water retention).

Recommended dose: 3–7g per day over a 30-day period. Creatine supplements should be taken in cycles, so you might take it daily for a month and then have a break. Taking a low dose like this daily for a month causes less water retention than 'loading up' for shorter periods with as much as 20g per day.

Hydroxy beta-methyl butyrate (HMB)

HMB is the resultant product of the breakdown of leucine, one of the body's essential amino acids. Playing an important role in muscle growth and repair, some research suggests that HMB supplementation can help with muscle and strength gains in novice strength trainers but not in more experienced participants. It is believed that HMB assists the body in minimizing protein breakdown following intense exercise.

Recommended dose: 1000mg per day.

Glucosamine sulphate

Glucosamine sulphate is a naturally occurring substance in the body which plays a role in keeping cartilage healthy and reducing 'wear and tear' on joints. Research has shown that supplementation may help with joint pain and osteoarthritis. For example, a study published in the *British Journal of Sports Medicine* found that 2000mg taken for twelve weeks

provided pain relief and improved function in 88% of subjects with knee pain. Other research suggests 1000–1500mg a day is sufficient and that the product works best when taken in conjunction with chondroitin (many supplements contain both so check the label).

Recommended dose: 1000–2000mg per day.

THE PERFECT PRE-AND POST-WORKOUT SNACKS

The goal of a preworkout snack is to provide some carbohydrate and protein calories, ideally along with hydration. Aim to eat it 30 minutes to an hour before your workout, rather than ten minutes before, to reduce the likelihood of it repeating on you. Try…yogurt, peanut butter on crisp breads, a banana, or an isotonic sports drink.

In the hours following your workout, taking in some protein and carbohydrate enhances recovery and helps promote an increased secretion of growth hormone (which helps to control body fat). But don't overdo it, a sports bar, half a tuna sandwich, or a pot of yogurt is sufficient.

As for during your session, it's only necessary to take calories on board if you are planning to do a challenging aerobic workout after your resistance session. If this is the case the easiest way of getting some ready fuel in is to drink an isotonic sports drink.

MAKING IT PART OF YOUR ROUTINE

Knowing how to strength train effectively is one thing but fitting it into your life – and your existing fitness routine – is quite another. Here's how your weights regime fits into the bigger picture.

OK, I know this is a book about strength training – but the truth is that a balanced exercise program – especially one with weight loss as its goal – needs to include both aerobic exercise and strength training (with flexibility work to keep muscles and joints healthy and supple). But how much is enough? And how hard do you have to work?

Creating a balanced program

We've already looked at how often and how hard to strength train in Chapter 5. So what about aerobic activity? The American College of Sports Medicine recommends three to five sessions per week of moderate- to vigorous-intensity activity, lasting 20–60 minutes, to improve aerobic fitness, while general health guidelines suggest we get a dose of 30 minutes moderate activity on most days of the week. If you think that 30 minutes is a lot bear in mind that the human body was designed to be a lot more active than that! Clocking up 30 minutes is actually a bare minimum for health benefits and, quite honestly, won't go a long way towards aiding weight loss if done in isolation.

In fact, the American College of Sports Medicine's *Position Stand on Weight Loss*, published in 2001, recommends building up to 200–280 minutes of activity per week for sustained weight loss – that's 40–60 minutes a day, five days a week. Sounds like a lot, huh? But this can – and should – consist of both 'daily activity' and structured workouts. For example, if you clock up the 30-minute daily dose on five days and throw in three more effortful 20-minute sessions on your bike or on the treadmill, then you are there. The daily dose doesn't even have to be completed all at once. In fact, its role is to replicate the more active lifestyles our ancestors used to live and can be made up entirely of routine daily activities like walking, climbing stairs, carrying and lifting, gardening, and doing household chores (see the box opposite for some ideas of where you could be more active).

You can easily get all the exercise you need – including your strength training – with three 50-minute sessions a week, coupled with general lifestyle activity on most days. In the gym you could follow your strength training session with a 30-minute swim or precede it with an aerobics class or treadmill run. That saves time while still allowing you to get the right balance of aerobic training and strength work. As we'll look at in a moment there is some feeling that concurrent strength and endurance work in the same session may reduce the benefits slightly, so if you have the motivation and time to train on separate days then you may gain slightly more – but in the greater scheme of things, the important thing is that you do it at all.

GETTING YOUR DAILY DOSE

Getting more active on a daily basis isn't about putting time aside for exercise, it's about using the time you have more effectively. It could be gardening, hosing down the garbage can, hand-washing the car, nipping to the shops on a bike, playing football with the kids, or chasing sticks with the dog. Really think about your daily lifestyle. Ask yourself if you are guilty of any of the following:

- Do you use a shopping cart when you could carry a basket?

- Do you park as close as you can to the supermarket/gym/station in the car park?

- Do you walk a dog and then stand still throwing a ball or stick?

- Do you walk to the closest sandwich shop at lunchtime?

- Do you sit up in the bleachers while the kids are swimming instead of going for a swim or power walk yourself?

- Do you stand still on escalators or wait for lifts?

- Do you drive to the station when you could walk?

- Do you email colleagues in the same building?

- Do you use a remote control for the TV or stereo?

- Do you pile things at the bottom of the stairs rather than taking them up at the time?

HOW MUCH EXERCISE DO I NEED FOR WEIGHT LOSS?

Scientists reporting in the *American Journal of Clinical Nutrition* stated that successful weight loss, maintained for a year, was achieved by either 80 minutes a day of *moderate*-intensity activity, or 35 minutes per day of *vigorous* activity. Higher intensity exercise will not only take up less of your time, it will also elicit more health and fitness benefits – but a mixture of strength training with some longer, more moderate aerobic activity and some shorter, sharper aerobic workouts will cover all bases without leaving you feeling burned out.

The weekly regime

Where does strength training fit in if you are already an aerobics addict, yogi, or runner? Not just in terms of finding the time to do both but also with respect to how to schedule both types of sessions to best effect. If you are already doing, or planning to do, aerobic exercise alongside strength training, you may be worried that you might reduce the effectiveness of what you are doing.

The general consensus about order of aerobic exercise and strength training is that concurrent strength and endurance training doesn't compromise endurance gains but *can* reduce strength gains. Since our focus is strength training this is an important consideration. One of the main factors seems to be the proximity of the two types of training. For example, following a tough treadmill run with resistance training may mean you aren't maximizing the benefits to be gained from the latter. Research shows that it is more effective to do the two types of exercise on different days. But if that doesn't fit into your real life, then in what order should you perform the two types of activity?

Results are conflicting. Some research found that strength development was not hindered when strength training immediately *preceded* endurance training, or when resistance training took place at least half an hour after endurance training. However, a recent study at Brigham Young University in Utah found that performing aerobic exercise *before* resistance work was more beneficial than the other way round – for two reasons. First, the resistance training made the treadmill run feel harder and, secondly, EPOC (the 'afterburn' calories that the body uses to restore systems to normal after exercise) was greatest when resistance work followed a treadmill run, thereby maximizing calorie expenditure. Keep the intensity of the preceding endurance activity moderate rather than high, too, if you don't want to compromise your strength training – a study from the University of Queensland found that high-intensity endurance exercise could inhibit performance in a subsequent resistance training session.

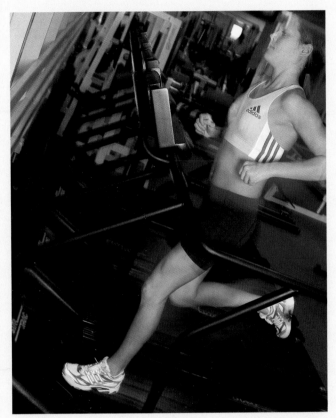

different adaptations caused by aerobic training and strength training, we have to ask, are circuits really an effective method of building strength, or less of a 'Jack of All Trades' and more 'Master of None'? This question was addressed by the Australian-based Fitness Network, who came up with the following recommendations for making circuits effective:

- Bear in mind that if you are doing 20–30 repetitions of an exercise, you are working not on strength but on muscular endurance. If you want to build strength, then intersperse sets of 6–12 challenging repetitions with 1 to 3-minute 'aerobic' recovery periods.

- If you are already familiar with strength training the overload provided by circuit training is unlikely to be sufficient to trigger further strength increases. In one study, it was shown that strength gains from circuit training for ten to twelve weeks were 5–25%, while the same period of time spent resistance training created improvements of 50–200%.

- The aerobic pay-off of circuit training isn't as great as standard aerobic training as the time spent at each station is short and the resistance work causes a buildup of lactic acid in the muscles therefore reducing the intensity at which you can work at the next station. Circuit training can improve aerobic capacity (VO_2 max) by 5–8% according to one study but conventional aerobic training is

On the circuit

Then there's another solution. Perform the two in the very same session. That, of course, is the premise behind circuit training. You do a strength training exercise, followed by a period of aerobic activity – each one being a 'station' on the circuit. The circuit might be completed two or three times in all. Some circuit training uses weight training machines, like the international franchise-based Curves gyms, while others use free weights and body weight for resistance.

But knowing what we know about the

likely to elicit far greater gains in the range of 10–35%.

- Ensure the circuit doesn't 'prefatigue' muscles with isolation exercises, such as triceps extensions or biceps curls, as this will limit the effectiveness of subsequent compound moves like squats, push-ups, and step-ups.

- The bottom line? If you enjoy circuit training and want a general workout – then go ahead. Additionally, if you are very mesomorphic and don't want to build muscle, this may be a good activity to utilize. But if your aim is to build strength, tone, and maximize weight loss, you are better off doing your aerobic exercise and strength work separately.

Fitting in other activities

It's all very well talking about strength and endurance exercise when the distinction between them is so clear. But what about, say, kickboxing, or rock climbing, or yoga? Where do these fit in?

Activities that are highly strength-dependent, like rock climbing, in which you are pulling and pushing your own body weight, are effectively a form of resistance training – so don't expect to do your weights workout on Saturday and not suffer on your wall climbing session on Sunday. However, activities that may leave your muscles a bit sore, like Spinning or kickboxing, aren't overloading the muscles in the same way as strength training (they are improving muscular endurance, not strength) so you could do them back to back without a problem.

Finally, activities like Pilates and yoga are good for building strength from within rather like the Foundation Workout. For inexperienced exercisers they are effectively like strength training but there will come a time when the challenge placed on your body, in terms of overload, won't be great enough to instigate further muscle development.

Keeping it balanced

When deciding whether you are ready for a strength training session there are two rules of thumb to follow: firstly, if your muscles are still sore from an activity it is best to delay your next strength training session. A bit of residual soreness is fine but if every move you make has you groaning in pain, forget it! Delayed onset muscle soreness (DOMS) is usually worst two days after the activity that caused it.

The second rule is the hard-easy rule. If you have worked really hard in one session (be it aerobic exercise or another type of activity) make your next workout a little more forgiving or take a rest day.

YOU KNOW WHAT?

A study showed that calorie expenditure and heart rate were significantly higher during exercises using the lower body or lower and upper body together, compared to just the upper body. So think below the belt, if making a tighter notch in it is your goal!

Staying on track

A lack of visible results is the prime cause of dropping out of exercise programs. Hopefully, that won't be your experience if you follow the advice in this book but that doesn't mean your resolve won't wobble occasionally. Here are some ways to stay on course…

Get practical

Do you keep missing your workout because the gym shuts so early? Or doesn't open early enough? If that's the case, swap gyms. Find somewhere that is more suited to your lifestyle. Maybe somewhere near to work rather than to home, for example. Or consider whether you could switch to home workouts, at least while you ride out a particularly busy period. Do you grab your kitbag and find it full of last week's smelly clothing and towel? Be organized by putting clean kit in your gym bag as soon as you get home from your last visit. Keep some spare kit at work or in the car as a back-up.

Beat boredom

If you are finding your workouts dull maybe it's time to find a new environment. Perhaps join a gym, so that you have the stimulation of other people around you, enlist a workout buddy (it always brings out your competitive streak!) or put some invigorating music on. New research from Brunel University saw up to an 18% improvement in adherence to exercise regimes with the help of the right music. You can also shake things up by adding new exercises to your repertoire, changing the structure of your workout, or

setting yourself a few goals. For example, pledge to deadlift 88lb in six weeks' time or hold a ball kneeling balance for a minute.

Re-focus

If you feel as if you are just going through the motions of your workout, you may have lost sight of what you are really doing it for. Think back to when you started strength training, and write down the reasons you started. Have you got closer to any of those goals? Is picking up your toddler easier? Can you lift heavy boxes that you previously had to ask your partner to shift? Do you walk to work now when you wouldn't have dreamed of doing so before? Give yourself some recognition for what you have achieved and make sure you know where you are heading next.

Make time

It's not so much that we don't have time to exercise, more that we don't schedule it in, simply hoping that we'll squeeze it in at some point. Realize that while exercise will take up minutes or hours of your week, the time spent doing it will enable you to use the rest of your day more productively. Not convinced? Well, studies show that exercise can improve mental function (such as decision making and problem solving skills), it can alleviate mild depression, and dissipate tension. What's more, when you exercise regularly, you actually become more stress-resilient so the day's problems will bounce off you rather than knock you down.

Find a role model

You might not want to look like one of those cover models on *Muscle & Fitness* magazine, but do you covet Nicole Kidman's shapely arms or Kelly Holmes' fantastic abs? Think of somebody who has a physique – or part of a physique – that you like and stick a picture of them on the fridge, or by your desk, to remind you that you need to keep on track if you want to reap visible results.

Pushing off a plateau

People often say that getting started with exercise is the most difficult bit, but I beg to differ! In the first few weeks the improvements come thick and fast, there's the novelty factor and you can't imagine why you didn't do it before. But a few weeks or months down the line perhaps you begin to feel as if you aren't making progress any more, the novelty has worn off, and it all feels a bit of a drag.

This is a very common experience and is probably the reason why more than half of those who take up exercise have given it up within six months. So what can you do to stay on course? Well, for starters, it's worth knowing that it is easier to make progress at the outset. This is because you are further away from your natural potential so you have more room for improvement. As you get fitter it is tougher to overload the body in order to instigate further changes. So it's not your imagination! But don't be disheartened by this truth. With what you have learned about manipulating your program, it shouldn't be too difficult to ring the changes and find a new way of challenging your body and making further progress.

Shake up your routine

Playing with different reps and sets isn't the only way to shake up your strength training regime. Here are a few other ideas…

Use unilateral movements

In other words, do exercises that you would normally do with both sides of the body or both limbs, with just one. For example, do a unilateral bench press, using alternate dumbbells, or use the leg press or leg curl machines with one leg at a time. Research shows that in free weight exercises unilateral work demands more core stability, so there's an added benefit, too.

Try metabolic circuits

This is a term used to describe a form of strength circuit-training. It is best performed with dumbbells or medicine balls – or just your body weight – and is most effective when lower and upper body exercises are alternated. (For example, a bench press is followed by a lunge.) The idea is to work swiftly – without compromising form – performing each exercise in the circuit for fifteen seconds, taking a 30-second rest afterwards. (Or, if you performed the exercise for 30 seconds, you'd take a one-minute rest – creating the same 1:2 work to rest ratio.) You then move on to the next exercise immediately. Once the circuit is complete, you repeat it – as many times as is appropriate for you.

Cut the rest

Shorter rest periods (less than a minute) won't maximize strength gains but they will stimulate the release of more growth hormone, contributing to fat loss.

Add instability

Instead of exercising on a weights bench, use an exercise ball to make your body work harder in order to stabilize itself. Or perform standing exercises on an unstable surface such as a core board or a balance pad.

Jump to it

Add power to your moves. Plyometrics is a system of exercise that makes use of the body's 'stretch-shortening' system. The notion is that the energy stored in the muscle allows for greater force to be produced rapidly. For example, instead of performing a squat with both feet on the ground you'd leap up off the floor, land back into a squat and go straight into the next one. However, this isn't a strategy to try until you are fairly experienced. I also recommend doing the moves initially without weight to get your body accustomed to it. If you want to give it a try do it at the start of your workout, when muscles are freshest, and aim for only a few repetitions.

Change the speed

A study published in the *Journal of Strength and Conditioning Research* from Appalachian State University in North Carolina also found that varying the speed of the exercise played a part in increasing strength and power in an eight-week program. Slow, controlled movements on some days were interspersed with fast, power-based moves on others.

Try a new technique

Yes! There is more than one way to lift a weight. Read on to find out about some of the popular methods...

Superslow training

In 'superslow' training, the weights are lifted and lowered very slowly (up to fifteen seconds per repetition) – the theory is that this forces more motor units to get a piece of the action. Some research has found much bigger strength gains from the superslow technique, compared to regular-speed training, but brand new research, published in *Medicine & Science in Sport & Exercise* found that faster training resulted in an 11% greater increase in strength than slow training did. The discrepancy in these findings once again goes to show that there is no single way to work that beats all the others. Throwing in the odd superslow session will do no harm and adds variety to your regime. But bear in mind that you will almost certainly have to drop the weight you use by 10–20% and perform fewer repetitions to reach fatigue.

Breakdown training

Aptly named, as this is no walk in the park. But breakdown training can be an effective way of blasting off a plateau, when you don't seem to be able to make further gains. The general idea is that you do your set as usual, with your standard weight, until you reach momentary muscle failure, then immediately decrease the resistance by 10–20% and continue to eke out as many reps as you can with this slightly lower weight. The premise behind this is that it forces the muscle to recruit more fibers to complete the work. Research at the South Shore YMCA in Massachusetts found that breakdown training worked well both for beginners and more experienced trainers. In eight weeks, beginners increased their weight load by an average of 25lb, compared to 18lb in a control group doing regular strength training. Experienced weight trainers saw significant improvements after just six weeks – performing a greater number of chin-ups and dips and lifting considerably more weight.

Eccentric training

Also called negative resistance training, this technique focuses only on the part of the muscle action in which the muscle is lengthening to control the movement initiated (for example, the lowering of the dumbbells in a bench press). Why would you do this? The theory is that muscles are stronger during the eccentric phase so working through this part of the movement can result in greater strength gains. As an example, you might get a partner to assist you in placing a barbell in your hands once you are in the top of a biceps curl position and then lower it with control. You can also do it sans partner. For example, you could lift a weight with both hands but lower it with just one. Research shows that the post-

BACK AND BICEPS WORKOUT

	1/3/06	5/3/06	8/3/06	10/3/06
Aerobic training	15 mins x-trainer	30 mins run	15 mins x-trainer	15 mins rower
Deadlift	4 x 4 66lb	4 x 5 66lb	4 x 5 66lb	4 x 6 66lb
Lat pulldown			3 x 8 88lb	
Assisted pull-ups	3 x 8 154lb	3 x 8 154lb		3 x 8 154lb
Seated row	3 x 10 66lb		3 x 10 66lb	
Single arm-row		3 x 8 33lb		3 x 8 33lb
Prone flye	2 x 8 9lb superslow	2 x 8 9lb superslow	2 x 8 9lb superslow	2 x 8 9lb superslow
Barbell curl				
Biceps curls	3 x 10 18lb	3 x 10 18lb	3 x 10 18lb	3 x 10 18lb

(3 x 8 154lb means 3 sets of 8 reps with a 154lb weight)

workout muscular aches (delayed onset muscle soreness or DOMS) you get from eccentric training is greater than from standard training, so be warned.

Supersetting

This is a time-efficient but challenging technique in which you pair up two exercises, usually those that work opposing muscle groups (such as the biceps and triceps), and perform an exercise for each with no rest in between. You only rest when you have finished the whole set. A variation on supersetting is 'compound' supersetting in which you alternate two exercises for the *same* muscle group with no rest between each one. So, you might team up bench presses with chest flys, for example. This is a very intensive way to train – but a great way to shake things up now and again, and has been shown to elicit size gains as well as strength.

Whatever technique or method you follow, don't do it forever. Variety is the secret to continued improvement – and interest.

The write way to keep on track

It is vital to keep a record of your strength training. It's impossible to remember how many reps and sets you did and what weight you used for every single exercise. A training log doesn't have to focus solely on your strength training either. It can include all your physical activity notes about what you ate and drank, your mood, your menstrual cycle… The only difference between a training journal for, say, running and a strength training log is

STRONG WORDS

PUT YOUR MIND WHERE YOUR MUSCLE IS

Take off that iPOD and transport your mind inside your muscles. Imagine the fibers shortening and lengthening and the blood flowing through them. Really focus on perfect posture and as you inhale, visualise the energy flowing to the muscle. Only close your eyes while you do this if you are securely situated on a fixed machine – otherwise, focus on your 'third' eye, a spot slightly above your eyes and in the middle.

that you need a lot more space for the latter. Most people use a simple notebook to keep track of their strength workouts or create blank sheets on the computer that they fill in. Don't forget to include information such as if you used a particular technique, such as superslow or supersetting, and, where relevant, comment on whether things worked well or otherwise. You may find it a bit tedious at first, to fill in the blanks after every workout, but once you see your weights climbing you won't be able to wait to fill in the next column!

AGES AND STAGES

Safe, effective strength training throughout life's ages and stages

Is strength training an activity you can benefit from at any age? You bet! But there are some precautions to take and some factors to be aware of when training during pregnancy, after giving birth, and during or post-menopause. This section gives you a little more information, but always consult your doctor if you are in doubt about whether strength training is appropriate.

Pregnancy – lifting for two

Internationally recognised guidelines from the American College of Obstetricians and Gynecologists (ACOG) state that exercise during pregnancy is not just safe but desirable. But does that include strength training? It does, but there are a couple of considerations to bear in mind. As with all types of training, pregnancy is a time to maintain what you already have rather than aim to achieve more. So put your goals aside for a few months and focus on holding on to the strength you have achieved thus far.

Here are a few other safety points to consider:

- Use slow, controlled movements because the effects of the hormone relaxin make your joints 'looser' and more liable to be injured.

- Stick to lighter weights to reduce the risk of injury.

- Don't hold your breath during exercises, which can increase blood pressure. Avoid the Valsalva maneuver (forcefully exhaling without actually releasing air which causes lower abdominal pressure similar to that of a bowel movement).

- Don't exercise in overheated environments and ensure you stay well hydrated.

- Avoid exercises that put you in a position where you could be at risk of dropping a weight on to your belly. So, for example, you would be safer to use the chest press machine rather than doing a dumbbell or barbell bench press.

- Beginning in the second trimester, avoid lifting weights while standing as the increased blood volume you have can cause blood to pool in your legs and cause dizziness or lightheadedness. Some experts believe that lying flat on your back decreases blood flow to the uterus too, so you may want to consider sticking with seated exercise.

- Be aware that some pregnant women are more prone to losing their balance since their center of gravity shifts forwards and upwards.

Don't exercise without medical advice if

- You are pregnant with twins or multiple babies.

- You have had previous miscarriages or premature births.

- You have hypertension (pregnancy-induced or otherwise).

- You have experienced bleeding.

STRONG WORDS

REASONS TO STAY STRONG

Half of all pregnant women experience back pain – probably due to the increased lordotic curve that results from pregnancy – but exercise to strengthen the abdominals prior to pregnancy will reduce the risk of being one of the unlucky 50%.

Exercise that strengthens the upper body – particularly in terms of keeping the upper and mid-back muscles strong – will also help avert the slumped posture many women adopt in pregnancy due to the increasing weight of their breasts and the changing center of gravity.

Recent research shows that physical activity may reduce the occurrence of gestational diabetes and pre-eclampsia by as much as 50% and 40% respectively.

- You feel any pain or discomfort from doing so.

- You don't feel confident about doing so.

Post-pregnancy

There are no hard and fast rules about when it is appropriate to resume exercise after pregnancy. ACOG recommends no physical stress for two weeks after delivery and not to return to full daily activities for a further four weeks. Additionally, if you have had a Cesarean delivery, you should avoid exercise for eight to ten weeks, to allow for full healing. Joint laxity, as a result of the relaxin, takes about twelve weeks to dissipate after pregnancy but that doesn't mean you can't begin some very gentle controlled exercises.

Take the floor

First on the list should be Kegel exercises. You will *not* regain strength or tone in the pelvic floor muscle without them. The easiest way to identify these muscles is to stop the flow of urine while you are on the loo, without clenching your buttocks. You basically need to do this movement every day for the rest of your life. Recent research suggests that you don't need to contract to your maximum; a slightly less than maximal contraction is more effective. Try 'the elevator' in which you contract upwards progressively over five levels – then release progressively over another five. Another good exercise to try is to imagine 'knitting' the walls of the vagina together – so you are squeezing together rather than pulling upwards.

Mummy's tummy

Over two-thirds of women experience an opening in the abdominal wall by the third trimester of pregnancy (known as diastis recti). It is vital not to do standard abdominal exercises post-pregnancy if this is the case, as it can prevent the gap from closing up. Even without diastis recti the rectus abdominis can stretch by as much as 8 inches during pregnancy while the transversus abdominis, which is responsible for providing core stability and protecting the lower back, will need to be strengthened and its

function restored. All women should wait until their post-birth check up before resuming standard abdominal exercises. Exercises for the abdominals that are safe to do before then are shown below.

On the pull

Finally, as you get to grips with being a new mum, try to focus your strength training efforts on the back of the body and pulling – rather than pushing – movements. Everything about motherhood – from nursing to changing nappies to putting baby in a car seat – involves forward movements and, without balancing work in the gym or with resistance, you may end up with a very 'forward' posture with hunched, rounded shoulders, tight chest muscles, a weak back, and flabby buttocks.

NAVEL TO SPINE CONTRACTIONS:

Inhale and, as you exhale, draw the navel gently into the spine. Hold for a few seconds without holding your breath. Build up to 20 second holds.

FRONT LYING ABDOMINAL RAISE:

Lie face down with your hands under your fore-head, head in line with the body. Keeping the rest of the body relaxed, inhale and, as you exhale, peel the navel off the floor, lifting the abdominals. Hold for 6 seconds, breathing freely, then relax. Do not lift the hipbones off the floor or contract the back.

PELVIC TILTS:

Lie on the floor with the knees bent, feet flat, and spine in neutral. Inhale and, as you exhale, draw the navel to spine and tilt the pelvis so the pubic bone curls towards you. Feel your back pressing lightly into the floor.

Menopause and strength training

Despite the huge emotive significance that menopause has in our society – the turning of the corner, the slippery slope towards old age, the passing of femininity – the menopause, put simply, is the signal of the end of reproductive potential. There is no longer enough of the hormones estrogen and progesterone to facilitate or sustain pregnancy. The average woman reaches menopause at 52 years old but the changes associated with the menopause can begin as much as a decade earlier. During this 'peri-menopause' stage, levels of the female hormones are depleting, influencing everything from mood to fat distribution and bone density and causing unwelcome effects like hot flushes and vaginal dryness.

For many women menopause goes hand in hand with weight gain and loss of lean muscle tissue. But research has not found any proof that weight gain is a direct result of menopause. In fact, one study found that women aged 42 to 50 gained the same amount of weight over that period whether or not they had been through the menopause, suggesting that lifestyle factors are more to blame. Peri-menopausal symptoms vary widely from woman to woman but there is a lot of evidence to suggest that regular exercise can soften the experience of the menopause. The Melpomene Institute found that physically active women rated their health through menopause much better than non-active women did. They were also less likely to suffer – or suffered less severely – with mental and physical symptoms of the menopause. Research shows that exercise is associated with a 55% decline in the frequency and intensity of hot flushes, for example.

So what about strength training? Well, the evidence suggests that resistance training can attenuate the loss of lean tissue, along with the accompanying decline in metabolic rate and the drop in levels of the muscle-building hormone testosterone. And a high lean body mass doesn't just look good – it is also associated with a high level of the type of estrogen known as estrone which is thought to protect against reproductive tissue cancers. A study from the University of Vienna put early post-menopausal women on an intense strength-training program for fourteen months. At the end of the study measures of strength, endurance, quality of life, and even bone mineral density had improved in women during the critical early post-menopausal years. Talking of which…

Aging bones and osteoporosis

The old 'use it or lose it' adage is often applied to muscle, but the same goes for bone density (the thickness and strength of the bone). The more you do sooner, the better. Peak bone mass – the maximum amount of bone you ever attain – occurs around the age of 20 and, from 30 or so, a slow decline begins. In the decades prior to menopause we lose 0.75–1% per year – but in the years following it bone density can plummet by as much as 5% per year which is why the bone-thinning condition osteoporosis – that causes

frailty, a high risk of fracture, and loss of height – affects one in two women over the age of 50 in the US.

According to the National Osteoporosis Foundation, regular weight-bearing exercise can reduce the accelerated rate of bone loss in post-menopausal women, even in the absence of hormone replacement therapy (HRT). Regular physical activity can reduce the risk of hip fractures by around 50%.

The best recipe for preventing osteoporosis is combining weight-bearing aerobic exercise with strength training. If you want proof, then consider that swimmers and cyclists, whose activity *isn't* weight bearing, have been found to have similar bone density as normally active people, while bodybuilders and gymnasts have bone density 30% higher than average.

A stronger skeleton

Why is strength training so good? Partly because, unlike running or jumping it can work the entire skeleton not just the lower half. You can actually target any muscle you like with specific exercises. The most common vulnerable sites for osteoporotic fractures are the spine, hip, and wrist. Also, because when muscles contract and pull on bone the force that the bone experiences causes it to increase its mass to better tolerate the contractions next time. The evidence suggests that resistance training successfully maintains or slightly improves hip and spine bone mass.

As I've said before, lifting light weights numerous times is not of much benefit – and this holds true in terms of bone health, according to expert Kerry Winters-Stone. It seems that high intensity is the name of the game – research shows that women who benefit as far as bone is concerned are working three sets with heavier weights.

If you already have osteoporosis you can still work with weights but you should do so under the guidance of your doctor. Start slowly, with lighter weights, in order to master the technique and movements involved. A weighted vest can be a good alternative to free weights for some exercises (for example, squats and lunges), as it keeps the weight close to the body and leaves the hands free. Alternatively, use resistance tubing so that you don't over-stress your joints or risk weight-related injuries.

Training and aging

Like it or not, with advancing age comes a natural decline in muscle mass and range of motion. The average adult loses 5–10% of muscle mass between the ages of 20 and 50. The strength of the back, leg, and arm muscles plummets by as much as 60% between the ages of 30 and 80, spinal extension range decreases rapidly, and ankle joints can lose half their range of motion between the ages of 55 and 85. With strength and muscle-mass loss comes a knock-on effect on metabolic rate and on our ability to do tasks that were once a cinch. Results from a large-scale epidemiological study found that 40% of the female population aged 55–64, 45% of women aged 65–74 and 65% of women aged 75–84 were unable to lift 10lb. It's a worrying prospect – but over and over again research shows that most of this decline occurs because we don't do anything to stop it. If we maintained muscle mass in the first place we'd offset the drop in metabolic rate, not gain excess body fat and continue to be active on a daily basis. A Scandinavian study published in the *International Journal of Sports Medicine* demonstrated that 70-year-olds who had lifted weights regularly for more than ten years had as much muscle as 28-year-olds.

Never too late

But what if the rot has already set in? Happily it isn't to late too do something to reverse the situation. Some classic research in a report in the *Journal of the American Geriatrics Society* showed that women aged 60–77 who strength trained for sixteen weeks could walk 20% faster, had gained a 50% increase in muscle strength and were able to sit or stand more comfortably for longer. Low bone mass, poor daily function, reduced muscle strength and postural instability are predictors of the risk of fracture in an elderly person, so any activity that can preserve strength and attenuate these risk factors is well worth doing. Once again, strength training takes center stage.

What's more, a study published in the *Journal of Applied Physiology* in 2005 found that, in older women, six months of resistance training resulted in a 4% increase in resting metabolic rate as well as a 9% increase in total daily energy expenditure (amounting, on average, to 177 calories per day). And the average age of the women was 72 years old!

Another important consideration is that, often, studies in which older adults are put on exercise programs don't result in them increasing their energy expenditure because they spontaneously decrease the amount of energy they burn the rest of the day. This has led some experts to suggest that gentler forms of activity like tai chi and walking are more suitable. But it is likely that this compensatory response is because the level of intensity of exercise in the study is too high, so the subjects are exhausted for the rest of the day. However, it appears from research that resistance training is less likely to have this effect than aerobic exercise. In fact, if the level of intensity is appropriate to begin with, and increased slowly but surely, it is possible that subjects could become *more* spontaneously active, as they have a better ability to cope with daily demands due to enhanced strength and aerobic capacity.

Exercise also reduces the risk of falls and accidents among older people through developing bone health and maintaining normal muscle strength and joint structure and function. Regular workouts can give older people a level of functional capacity associated with people ten to fifteen years younger.

Exercising safely in later life

- Warm up thoroughly. Levels of elastin (the stretchy component in connective tissue) deteriorate with age making muscles and tendons more injury-prone.

- Think about functional exercises rather than

STRONG WORDS

IS STRENGTH TRAINING SAFE AFTER BREAST CANCER?

According to a study from the University of Pennsylvania in 2005 the answer is yes. A randomized controlled trial assessed the safety and effects of twice-weekly weight training among recent breast cancer survivors. Those who strength trained showed increases in lean mass as well as significant decreases in body fat and a self-perceived better quality of life.

about honing in on single muscle groups. For example, a squat is much more akin to daily activities than is a leg extension. A shoulder press overhead is more useful than a triceps kickback…

- Allow yourself longer to recover between sessions.

- Heed the ACSM guidelines for strength training for older adults. These recommend 10–15 repetitions for adults 50–60 years of age or older.

- Watch your protein intake. Studies show that many older adults are not eating enough protein and, if you are strength training, this is even more important. The ACSM guidelines suggest 1.0–1.25g of high-quality protein per kg (2.2lb) of body weight per day.

Directory

You've got the book, you've done the workout – now you want the t-shirt, and the shoes, and the exercise ball! You should find everything you need to help you get stronger on these pages…

Equipment

Bowflex
A home gym machine on which you can perform over 60 exercises, based on rods and pulleys.
(888) 346 7068 or www.bowflex.com

Proform
Home aerobic machinery such as treadmills and elliptical trainers.
(888) 742 0128 or www.proform.com

Life Fitness
A comprehensive and reliable range of weight-training equipment and aerobic machines.
www.lifefitness.com

Power Systems
Sports and Fitness equipment.
www.power-systems.com

Nautilus
An extensive range of strength-training products, from weight stations, racks, benches, and bars to dumbbell sets,
www.nautilus.com

The Physical Company
A huge range of exercise mats and balls, medicine balls, resistance tubing, core stability equipment, and a wide range of free weights, including dumbbells and barbells.
01494 769 222 or
www.physicalcompany.co.uk

Omni Fitness Equipment
A massive range of products from weight benches to yoga mats, treadmills to core boards, mini trampolines to body bars.
www.omnifitness.com

I don't know what dumbbells to buy – any advice?
Why not start off with a set of dumbbells in different weights? You can get a set of three different weights quite cheaply and these will give you more scope than just having one set. Alternatively, you could invest in dumbbells on which you attach weight plates so that the amount you lift can be varied quite significantly. The best thing to do, if you don't have the opportunity to try a few different weights at the gym, is to go to a sports store where you can actually see and pick up what is on offer.

I like…
One of the best bargains around is the V-Fit trio of dumbbells from Argos, available for home delivery (www.argos.co.uk). Two at $3^{1}/2$lb, two at $6^{1}/2$lb and two at 11lb give a beginner plenty of scope.

What essentials should I have in my gym bag?

What gets you through a workout varies from person to person. But everyone should have a drinks bottle to hand, to ensure that you stay hydrated while you train. You will almost certainly need a gym towel, too — not only to wipe off your sweat but also to protect your skin from other people's. The Marsupial towel is a great version that has a Velcro pocket on it for locker keys and iPODs (www.marsupialtowel.com). The other essential, in my opinion, is a training log and pen so you can jot down your reps, sets, and weight lifted at the time of training. And finally, a pair of weight-training gloves, if you are precious about your hands! Lifting weights will eventually cause hard skin to build up below your fingers if you don't wear gloves.

I like…

A new take on elastic resistance, called the Digiband. Thanks to the Digiband's "powermarks," little oval-shaped icons with a weight printed in them, you can keep tabs on how much weight you're pushing or pulling. When you stretch the band enough to make the oval turn into a circle you are working at the resistance stated. Cheap, lightweight, and available in three strengths, it is available from www.proactive-health.co.uk.

Clothing

What should I wear to workout in?

You can wear anything that is loose and comfortable (especially if you are exercising at home!) Avoid clothes that are too baggy or flowing as they may get caught in machinery – and besides, they don't allow you to keep tabs on your body position and technique. Breathable fabrics are best for wicking away sweat from the body and allowing it to evaporate – look for brand names Coolmax, Climacool, and Dri-fit.

Adidas

Performance-orientated clothing, accessories, and footwear.
(800) 982 9337 or www.adidas.com

Casall

Stylish activewear, underwear, and accessories for fitness.
www.casall.co.uk

Activa Sports

A sports bra specialist.
(888) 566 7792 or www.activasports.com

New Balance

Clothing, footwear, and accessories.
(800) 622 1218 or www.newbalance.com

Nike

Clothing, footwear, and accessories including weight-training gloves.
(800) 344 6453 or www.nike.com

GirlMax Sports

Women's active ware.
www.girlsportsbrand.com
(877) 392 4263

Sweaty Betty

Own-brand and other high-end brands of sportswear, footwear, equipment, and accessories for women.
www.sweatyBetty.com

What sort of shoes should I wear?

A pair of cross-sneakers, with adequate support, stability, and cushioning is fine for strength training. If you are going to be combining resistance training with high-impact aerobic exercise at the gym, however (such as running or aerobics), then you are better off investing in shoes designed for your particular activity and wearing them for your gym workout. Running shoes are not ideal for aerobics or kickboxing type classes as they don't have any lateral support and lack forefoot cushioning.

Supplements

With supplements, you tend to get what you pay for – cheap brands are often less effective and don't contain sufficient doses of the active ingredients. Buy supplements from a reputable source and check the dosage and concentration of the relevant ingredient. Here are some good places to start…

www.highfive.co.uk (for own brand energy, protein, and creatine supplements).

www.thenutricentre.com (for a variety of brands and a useful search facility).

www.vitaminshoppe.com (for a variety of vitamins, herbs, and sports nutrition).

www.solgar.co.uk (for own-brand vitamin and mineral supplements).

Useful organizations

USTrainer
By searching this national database of qualified, experienced personal trainers you should be able to find the right person to help you get the basic techniques of strength training correct and keep you motivated.
www.ustrainersearch.com

National Strength and Conditioning Association
A US-based body that conducts extensive research into the effects of strength training, maintains a comprehensive website, publishes journals, and offers courses for becoming a qualified strength coach.
www.nsca-lift.org

www.strongwomen.com
Run by Dr Miriam Nelson, a leading researcher in women's health and the role of strength training, this US-based site has some useful tips and articles.

Recommended reading

An Action Plan for Osteoporosis
(Kerri Winters-Stone, Human Kinetics)

The Complete Guide to Post-natal Fitness
(Judy deFiore, A&C Black)

The Weight Loss Bible
(Joanna Hall, Kyle Cathie)

Strength Training Anatomy
(Frederic Delavier, Human Kinetics)

Glossary

Aerobic Literally means "with oxygen," but usually refers to exercise that relies on aerobic metabolism

Atherosclerosis Accumulation of fat on the artery walls resulting in a narrowing of the vessels and risk of heart attack or stroke

Anaerobic In the absence of oxygen (although this is never entirely the case). But usually refers to short, sharp efforts in exercise, in which energy cannot be supplied fast enough through aerobic metabolism. Strength training is an example

Basal metabolic rate The rate at which your body ticks over at rest, usually measured following a 12 hour fast and a night's sleep

Body composition The ratio of body fat to lean tissue

Body mass index A method of estimating and classifying body composition based on weight and height

Bone mineral density A measure of the amount of bone mineral content

Cardiac output The amount of blood pumped from the heart in one minute

Cardiorespiratory Relating to the heart and lungs

Cardiovascular Relating to the heart and blood vessels

Cartilage A tough connective tissue found throughout the body

Concentric A muscular contraction that takes place while the muscle is shortening

Compound An exercise that uses multiple muscle groups

Contraction Muscle pulling to create force

Core stability Control and appropriate strength and function of the stabilizing muscles throughout the body. Often refers specifically to those of the abdominals and back

Diastolic The lower part of a blood pressure reading, representing the phase during which the heart muscle relaxes

Eccentric A muscular contraction that takes place while the muscle is lengthening

Engage To consciously recruit a muscle

Extensor A muscle that straightens a joint

Fast-twitch fiber A type of muscle fiber that reaches maximum tension very fast but also fatigues quickly

Flexor A muscle that bends a joint

Glycemic Index A classification of the effect of a carbohydrate food on blood sugar levels

Glycogen The body's storage form of carbohydrate, stored in the liver and in muscles

Heart rate The number of times the heart beats per minute

Hypertrophy A growth in physical size of a muscle

Isometric A muscular contraction in which the muscle stays the same length

Lean body mass The proportion of the body made up of non-fat tissue (including muscle, connective tissue, and bone)

Ligament Connective tissue that joins bone to bone

Periodization A planned training program consisting of different phases or cycles with a specific purpose and progression towards a specific goal

Progressive overload The principle that states that in order for the body to continue getting fitter, the workload needs to be gradually but consistently increased

Prone Face down

Resting heart rate The number of times the heart beats per minute at rest

Sarcomere The functioning unit within a muscle fiber

Slow twitch fiber A type of muscle fiber that is fatigue resistant but slow to reach maximal power. Best suited to low power, long duration activities.

Somatotyping A system of classification of body types by shape and proportions

Submaximal Below maximum effort or intensity

Supine Face up

Synovial fluid The sticky substance found in joints which adds cushioning and lubricates joint structures.

Systolic The top part of a blood pressure reading, which represents the phase during which the heart muscle contracts

Total Energy Expenditure The amount of energy used in a day, including resting metabolic rate

Tendon Connective tissue that joins bone to muscle

Valsalva Maneuver A technique in which one increases the pressure within the abdominal and chest cavity by forcibly breathing out while keeping the throat closed to trap and pressurize air in the lungs

Index

Acknowledgements

My greatest appreciation goes to Pat Fox, strength and conditioning specialist at the Human Performance Center, South Bank University – not just for his valuable feedback and contributions to the text but also for showing me how to kneel on a balance ball and perfect my deadlift! Sincere thanks also to Sarah Connors, from the Back on Track Sports Injury Clinic in London, for her time and input in developing the Foundation Workout – true strength comes from within…

Adidas and Casall provided the fantastic clothing for the photo shoots, while the Physical Company and Gaiam kindly loaned us a wealth of fitness equipment and gadgets. Rachel Fradgley, Jill Christie, Juliet Murrell, and Lulu Valentine did a sterling job being supermodels and Guy Hearn took the fantastic photographs. Thanks to you all.